The Illustrated Guide To Threesome Sexual Positions

How To Take Sex To The Next Level

by C.W. Pollard

Overunity Publications

First Edition: 2012

ISBN 978-1475015201

Although the author and the publisher believe that the included information is accurate and useful, nothing contained in this publication can be considered professional advice on any legal or accounting matter. You must consult a licensed attorney or accountant if you want professional advice that is appropriate to your particular situation.

Introduction

In this book, we are going to explore a variety of threesome sexual positions. Before we do this, I want to make sure that we are all on the same page concerning threesome sex.

First of all, in the right situation, threesomes can be a lot of fun. There is an air of play that manifests itself in a threesome that does not necessarily appear when a couple is making love. There is a lot of sexual exploration and usually a lot of laughing and giggling in a threesome.

Threesomes also have a way of capturing our imaginations and our fantasies as well. A man will fantasize about being with two women. A woman will fantasize about what it is like to be with two me. Both sexes fantasize about what it is like to be with a partner from each gender at the same time. If you have had a threesome you probably had fun. If you haven't you are most likely curious. Either way, whoever you are, there is a good chance that a threesome is somewhere in your fantasy wishes.

The last point i want to make before we start actually exploring how to make love with two partners at the same time, is that a threesome, by nature, is less natural than one on one sex. Now, this is not a moral judgment. It is simply a statement of fact. When a man and a woman make love, there is a biological coupling that takes place. This coupling, physically speaking, has been designed and refined to work ergonomically for a million years or more. Essentially, Mother Nature has designed a man and a woman to fit together so the act is natural.

Threesome sex is different. Three people are not designed to fit together with no parts being left over. Many of the sexual positions that are discussed in this section will seem a touch artificial. Well, they are. Palm trees in Minnesota are artificial too, but that doesn't mean you can't enjoy them.

So as we go three these positions together, keep in mind that there may be some left over parts. Somebodies clit or cock may not be getting attention. That's OK. Threesome sex, just like one on one sex is about sharing, taking turns and having fun.

Now, let's get to the fun stuff.

A Discussion Of The Difficulty Rating System Used

All of the positions in this book are achievable. Nothing here will push the human body beyond it's limits. However, all the positions are rated from easy to moderate to hard and I want to quickly define what those mean, in the context of this work.

Easy - An easy sexual position will require no work from the couple to maintain it. Once it is entered into nobody will have to work to keep their balance. There is no chance of falling over and the position is perfectly comfortable to everyone involved. These positions would be described as very natural sexual coupling positions.

Moderate - A moderately difficult sexual position involves more than this. It is going to take a little work from the couple. At least one member of the couple is going to need to work to maintain their balance. There is a chance of falling over onto the bed in the heat of passion. These are the positions you need to work a little bit at and may push parts of the body in ways it was not meant to bend, although not uncomfortably so.

Difficult - Difficult sexual positions, as far as this book is concerned are the positions that the couple needs to work together to maintain. They must work as a couple and coordinate their efforts. He must support her while she assumes a body form that is hard to keep going, or vice versa. There are not many of these positions in this book. However, these ones can be especially fun and the teamwork needed to make them happen only brings a couple closer together.

A Few Word On Female Orgasm For The Gentlemen

In this book, each sexual position lists whether or not it is good for female orgasm. I want to write a few words discussing this.

First, of all I want to make sure that you, the reader, understands that I am only referring to clitoral orgasms. This is the type of orgasm that any woman can have, provided that her clit is stimulated correctly and she is relaxed enough.

Vaginal orgasms and the G-spot fall into the realm of the Sasquatch. They may very well be real, I will not argue that point. However, medical science has yet to demonstrate conclusively whether or not they are. Since this is the case, I am not going to focus on them. The clitoris is real, very easy to find, and very easy to use to make a woman orgasm. Just about 100% of sexually active women will have masturbated via their clit and I am sure that they will agree with me.

Now, all of the pussy eating positions in this book can be used to give a woman an orgasm. It simply requires stimulating her clit with your mouth. This is sometimes trickier that others, and those positions discuss that in detail. However, if you want to make a woman orgasm, this is your first place to start.

For those of you looking to learn more about pussy eating, please consult my other work <u>The Secret Art Of Eating Pussy : Tips & Tricks To Please Her Every Time</u> (ISBN 978-1463655631) available via all online retailers.

For the intercourse positions that list that they are good for female orgasm, you really have three choices and I am going to tell you about both. Both of these options involves direct clitoral stimulation during intercourse.

The easiest and most basic way to stimulate the clitoris (I'm going to assume you know where it is) is manually with fingers. This can be done either by her or by her lover and it is up to the couple to decide which is best given the position.

Either way, you should stimulate her clitoris using your index and middle fingers, as shown in the picture below.

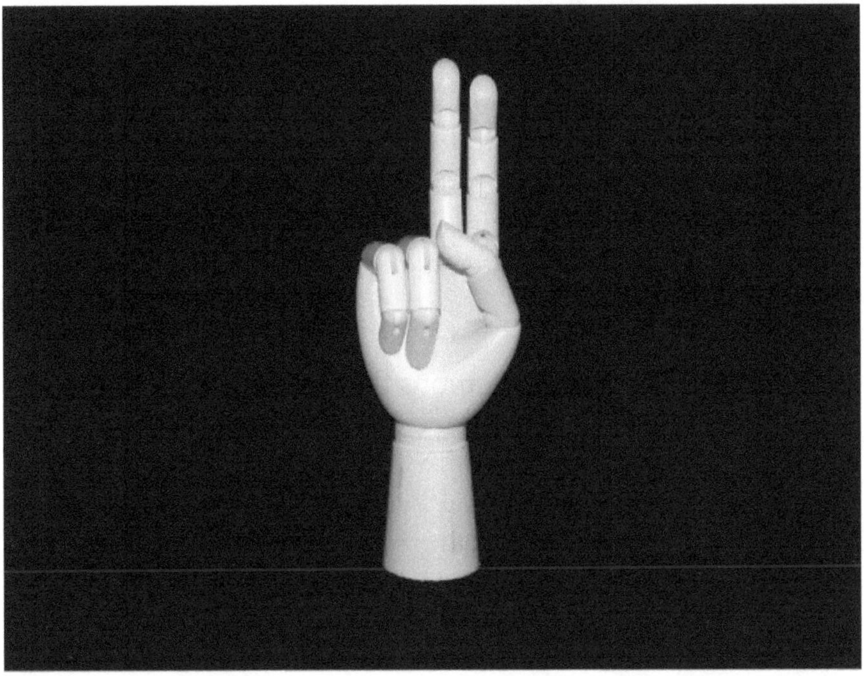

Men, if you are doing the fingering, make sure to lick your finger before your touch her pussy. I mean really lick it. Get it nice and wet with saliva, this will make sure everything is nice and lubricated and there won't be any chaffing.

Find her clit, and position your fingers so her clit is sitting right between your two fingers. Keep them together. Now, apply gentle pressure to her clit. Start light!!! You can always increase pressure as things heat up.

Start by rubbing her clit (this is all while you are inside her) in small circular motions. Like I said, start gentle and go from there. You can always get rougher and go faster. Start slow and gentle.

While you are doing this, apply gentle pressure into her vagina with your cock. You don't have to really fuck her at this point. It is more than enough that you are inside her. Just move it in and out a little bit while you are doing what I said with you fingers. With a little luck she will be cumming in no time.

Now some of the sexual positions that I describe may be a little tight and you may not have the full range of motion you need to give her an orgasm with your fingers. There are also other issues like the man being too aggressive and actually hurting her clit or his hand can cramp up. All of these are a problem.

Well, modern technology has come up with a solution that you cannot afford to ignore. Meet the "bullet" style vibrator. These very small vibrators address all of these problems. They are small enough to get in the tightest squeezes (no pun intended) and they never cramp up. They will provide constant, uninterrupted stimulation to her clit while intercourse is going on. They are a tool that should be in the nightstand table for any sexually satisfied couple.

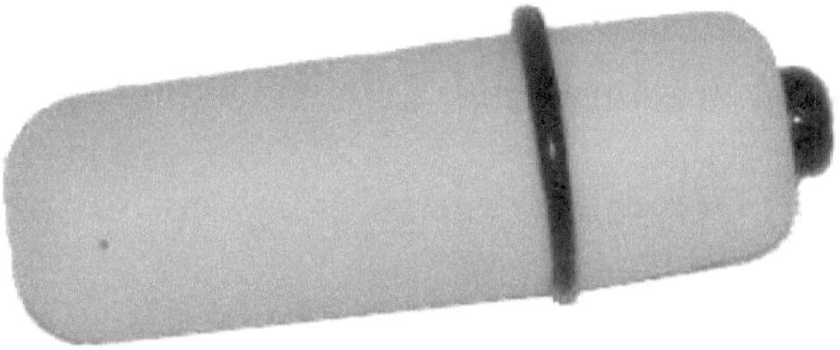

Now, I have mention that you, the man, can finger her or stimulate her with a vibrator. However, we live in enlightened times and I want you to know that she can do it too. There is absolutely nothing wrong with her fingering her clit or using a vibrator on her while the two of you are having sex. In fact, you should look at it as a good thing. For one, she is open enough to do that in front of you. Two, it is really sexy to watch. Three, it will make her cum and that is really the goal here. Lastly, sex will be more fulfilling, wilder when it happens and will happen more often.

Remember, the goal is a rosy cheeked, sexually satisfied woman. Nothing more, but certainly nothing less. You just want it to happen. How it happens is really just a minor detail.

Any And All Twosome Positions Still Apply

Threesomes are any sexual act that involves three people. Now, this does not mean that all three people have to be involved in the act of sex (penetrating, licking, sucking, etc.) for it to count as a threesome. In the threesomes that I have been involved in, there were plenty of times where another partner and I, or my other two partners were involved in a sex act, and the third merely watched.

This has a couple of implications that may not be apparent at first glance. I want to illustrate these to help make sure that any menage a trois that you may participate in have a better chance of being the fun, wild, sex, spontaneous fantasy that you hope they will be.

First, I am going to tell you right here in plain English, that it is OK if not everyone is involved with 100% of the action, 100% of the time. Sometimes, there just isn't room. Sometimes, someone has been hard fucking for an hour, they're all sweaty and the need a break. Sometimes someone has just ejaculated for the third time in a short period and their cock is as limp as al dente linguini. It happens. No worries. Take a load off, relax, and enjoy the show.

Second, any sexual position that involves two people has a place in a threesome. Don't just rely on the positions in this book. Two people can easily go at it and everyone can have a great time in a threesome. Remember, watching is a huge part of the fun. Sitting back and watching your partner in the act is a huge thrill.

This means that you should have more than a basic repertoire of twosome sex positions at your disposal. Not to toot my own horn, but my first book on sexual positions (An Illustrated Guide To Practical Sexual Positions :Everything You Need To Know For Wild Monkey Sex ISBN 978-0983927365) will get you well on your way to position proficiency.

Another reason that twosome sex is relevant to threesome sex is that some threesomes don't involve overlap. It may be more comfortable for the people in the threesome (usually partners of the same gender) to simply share a partner back and forth. This means that a woman can take turns having twosome sex with two men, or vice versa. This is still a sex act involving three people, and still counts, it will just involve a lot of twosome sex.

This type of threesome will often happen when a trio first gets together to fuck, however, as people become more comfortable, more warmed up and more horny, the acts will often intermingle into full on menage a trois, everyone involved sex.

Threesomes Are A Much About Watching As Doing

Anyone who has never had a threesome may easily overlook this truth. Watching people have sex can be as much of a thrill and as much fun as having sex yourself. This is not to overlook that it is a huge turn on as well.

Threesomes offer ample opportunities for the voyeur in all of us. If two members of the party should be engaged in some vigorous lovemaking, there is nothing wrong with kicking back and just watching the fun. There is nothing wrong with imagining yourself to be part of the action while you play with yourself either. Do what comes naturally and enjoy. Remember, in a threesome there are few rules. Find what you enjoy and indulge.

Make Sure Everyone Is Included

When you first engage in a threesome, there is a danger that you may not be aware of. I am going to point this out to you and talk about a few ways that you can avoid the problems that it can create.

This danger is that in a threesome, two of the partners focus solely on each other and ignore the third person. This is all too common. Say for example, a woman brings home a girlfriend for her and her husband to play with. The husband gets really excited and focuses on the novelty of the girlfriend and ignores his very generous, sexy wife. Well, in this situation, what do you think will happen? The wife will feel slighted, get angry, maybe even resentful and threesomes will be a thing of the past, if the couple is even still on speaking terms.

This is a classic rookie mistake. The example of vilifies a horny husband, but the same can be true in any threesome pairing. A horny young woman, eager to experiment in bisexuality may focus on her new female lover, or can just as easily get drunk on the novelty of a second cock. Well, again, her other lover will feel slighted and hurt feelings arise and from there, nothing but problems.

All of you need to work together to make sure that everyone is feeling included.

First rule for preventing these problems is to make sure that everyone is taking turns. Sharing should be a dominant theme in any successful threesome. If you have been riding a cock for a while, make sure you stop, and offer the chance to your other lover. If you have lavished your attention on one of your lovers for a while, make sure that you give some to the other. You should always be aware of how much time you are spending with your lovers in a threesome and be giving to both.

Taking on the role of the director is another way to make sure that everyone is feeling the love and having a good time. Don't be afraid to say something like "Let's double team him" or "You go down on her while I kiss her." Trust me people will appreciate this sort of direction in a threesome. Most people are just waiting for someone to play this role and tell them what to do and how to do it. (As a side benefit, assuming this role is the easiest way to get to see everything you want. If you want to watch your girlfriend go down on another guy, just tell her. Most likely, she will appreciate the go ahead and you get to live out a fantasy.)

Remember, another name for a threesome is "menage a trois" this literally means "house of three" in French. Think about that. Three equal partners. Not one partner joining a couple. Focus on equality and free sharing in a threesome and you will have a good time and many more in your future. If you fail to abide by these words, you will risk never getting oral sex from two lovers at the same time again. Remember that as you study the positions listed on the pages that follow.

Coming & Going

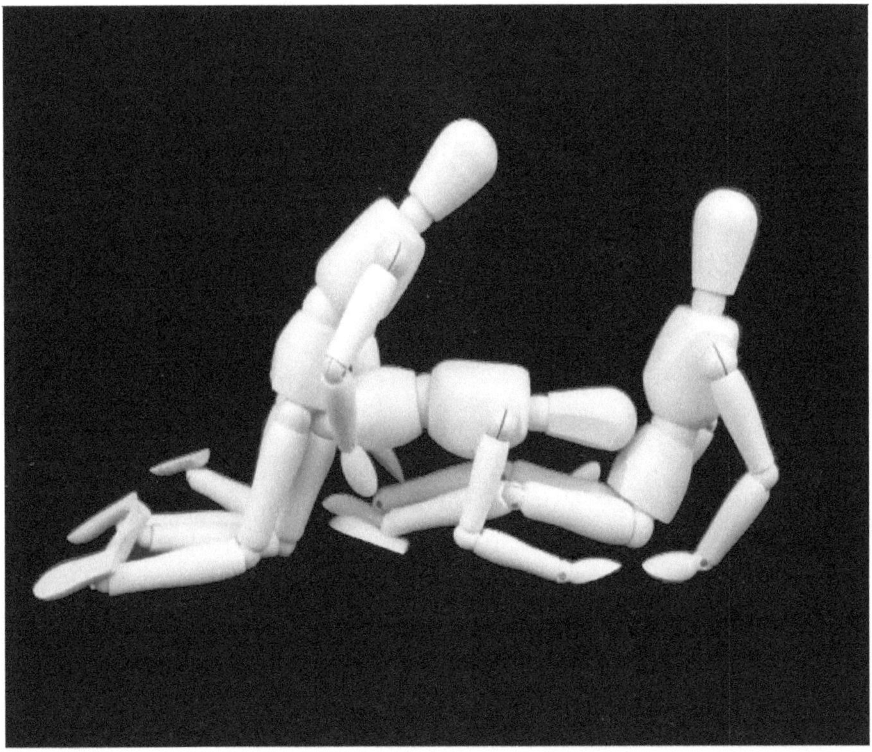

Position Description:

The woman places herself into a four point stance. One of her male lovers then takes a position behind her and penetrates her. Her other lover then places himself in front of her so she can give him oral sex.

Ease Of Position: Easy

Depth Of Penetration: Deep

Good For Female Orgasm? Yes

Downsides:

The woman is placed in the position of having to keep a lot of stuff going at once. She must support herself while one lover fucks her, while at the same time keeping a blowjob going for the other. This can often be too much and she may loose concentration. If she does, it is the guy getting the blowjob that loses out. However, if that happens, he needs to be a patient gentleman and wait until her focus returns.

Upsides:

For the woman, all of the attention is on her. She has two lovers who are eager and waiting for her attentions. This can make her (secretly of course) feel sexy and desirable. These are great positives to her self esteem. Additionally, many men love the idea of having sex with two lovers at once, well, women are no different. She really gets her cake and gets to eat it too in this position.

Notes On This Position:

This is definitely one of the basic threesome sex positions. Any threesome involving two men should take full advantage of this position. It is fun for all. She is having sex with two lovers at once and the men each get to watch her having sex at the same time. A definite visual and physical stimulation extravaganza.

I did mention patience earlier and that is worth noting. In this position, it is possible for the woman to become distracted and unable to focus on one of her lovers for a moment. If this happens, the guys need to be patient and wait. They can also take turns and switch positions to help alleviate this concern.

Coming & Going With Reacharound

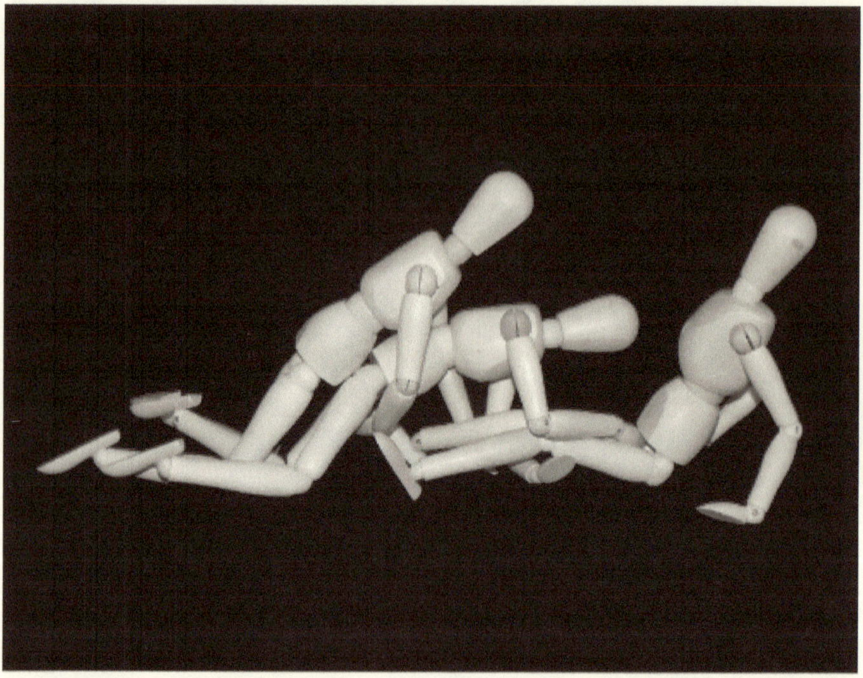

Position Description:

This position is a modification of the Coming & Going position that was just described. However, in this modified version, the penetrating partner (the one fucking from behind) reaches around and plays with what is found. If he is penetrating a woman either vaginally or anally he can no play with her clitoris. If he is penetrating a man anally, he is more than able to manually stimulate this lover to orgasm.

Ease Of Position: Easy

Depth Of Penetration: Deep

Good For Female Orgasm? Yes

Downsides:

For the lover in the middle, this position may push them towards sensory overload. They are being penetrated at the same time they are being stimulated to their own orgasm still at the same time they are orally stimulating yet another lover orally. This is a lot of balls in the air (no pun intended). It is easy for one to get dropped and for one lover to feel a little shortchanged or like an after thought. If this is the case, be a grown up and just wait your turn.

Upsides:

For the lover in the middle, this position may push them towards sensory overload. No, that is not a typo. That is the same sentence. It's true that what can be a little bad can also be a huge turn on. This position is one of those. If the lover can take the sensory stimulation , this position can offer them rarefied heights of ecstasy.

Notes On This Position:

If the lover in the middle is a woman, the penetrating partner should slow down the penetration and make sure it's not too deep. This will help her achieve her orgasm.

If, on the other hand, the penetrated partner is a man, the vigorous penetration combined with the handjob will be more than welcome and will make his orgasm all the more intense.

Pussyeating Doggystyle

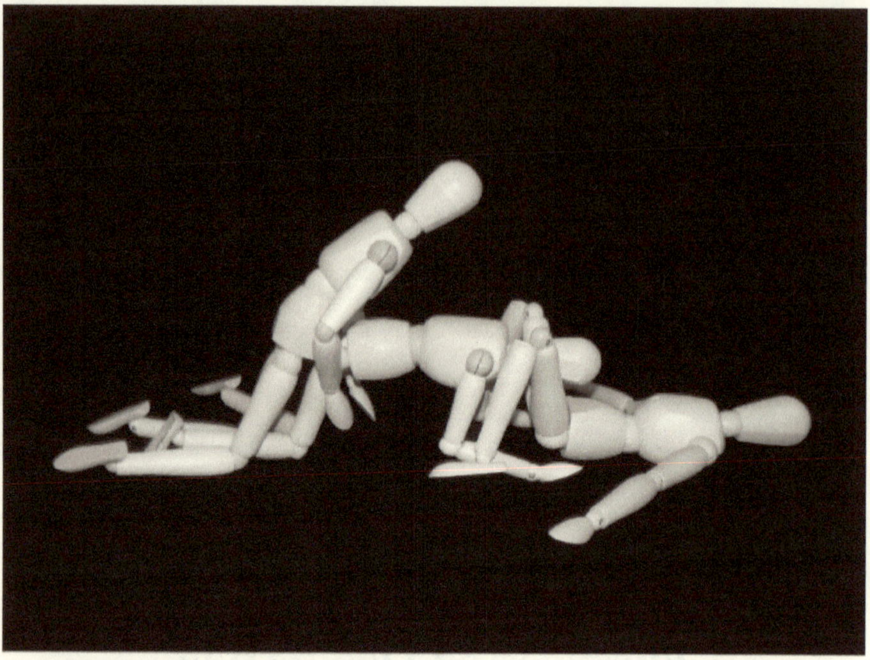

Position Description:

In this position, one woman lies on the bed in the standard pussyeating position. Another woman then assumes a four point stance and begins to eat her pussy. Lastly, the man comes up behind the woman in the four point stance and enters her.

This is generally a position for a threesome involving two women, although a man can play the part of the middle person.

Ease Of Position: Easy

Intimacy Level: Moderate

Wild Spontaneous Level: Moderate

Depth Of Penetration: Deep

Good For Female Orgasm? Yes

Downsides:

The same issues exist with this position as with the last one. The middle woman is put in the position of having to keep a lot of things going at one time. Eating a pussy can be tricky at times. You need to focus and be consistent. That's hard enough without being fucked at the same time. If you throw that in the mix, concentration and focus are going to go down. That being said, the pussyeating in this position may not be ideal.

Upsides:

The woman in the middle is getting a lot of stimulation and this time from both genders. She gets to be face to face with a woman in a very intimate way, while at the same time getting some very serious attention from a gentleman as well.

Notes On This Position:

For the female orgasm marks, I put that this position is good. That is technically true. The man or middle woman can easily stimulate the middle woman's clitoris and the woman having her pussy eaten is obviously getting stimulation there. That all being said, getting everything lined up so the women can actually cum, is harder than it may seem. Don't get frustrated if it isn't perfect right out of the gate.

With threesomes, it is often better for both lovers to focus on one of the women (think one giving oral sex and the other making out) at a time to make her cum. There is less timing that needs to work out and the sensation of two sets of hands all over a woman's body, focusing on her pleasure, often makes her orgasm a speedy affair.

Pussyeating Doggystyle With Reacharound

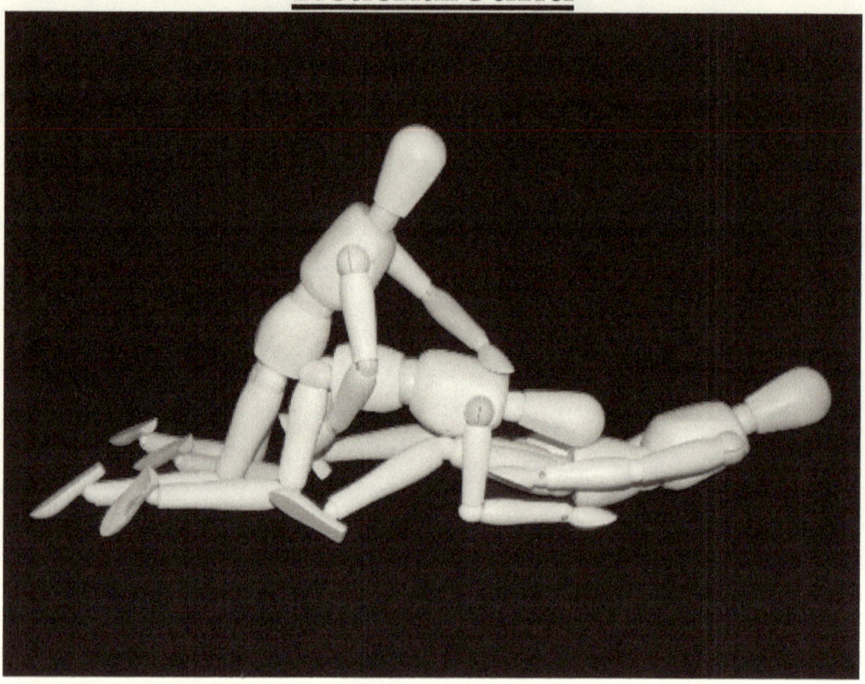

Position Description:

This position, like Coming & Going With Reacharound, is a modification of an existing position, the Pussyeating Doggystyle.

Again, in this position, the penetrating partner reaches around and stimulates either the clit or penis of the person they are fucking. The person who is getting fucked, continues to eat the pussy of the woman in front of them.

Ease Of Position: Easy

Depth Of Penetration: Deep

Good For Female Orgasm? Yes through intercourse or through pussyeating.

Downsides:

Just like the Coming & Going with Reacharound, there is a lot going on for the person that is both getting fucked, having their clit or cock stimulated and trying to give oral sex to a woman.

This position is even harder in that pussy eating tends to need to be much more precise to be effective in orgasm. This may just be too much to keep track of.

Upsides:

Again, like the Coming & Going with Reacharound, the person in the middle of this sexual act is nearing pleasure overload. They're getting it all and they are in the middle of everything. This can be very intense stimulation if they can relax enough to enjoy it all and not go mad before they cum over and over again.

Notes On This Position:

Since the person that is getting fucked is trying to eat pussy at the same time, a few words should be said about this. This may just bee too much to keep going in order to successfully eat another woman's pussy to orgasm. With pussy eating you need to be both consistent and precise and work in harmony with the woman who is getting the oral sex. This may be too much for this position. Getting fucked at the same time has a way of knocking you off course and causing stimulation to be inconsistent.

This is not to say that this position cannot be fun. It may be that the pussy eating just needs to stay foreplay, non-goal oriented. She can cum later, or even before, or the two ladies (if that applies to your threesome) can take turns and switch positions until everyone has had their fill. Remember, successful threesomes always have flexible partners who make it work.

One Then The Other

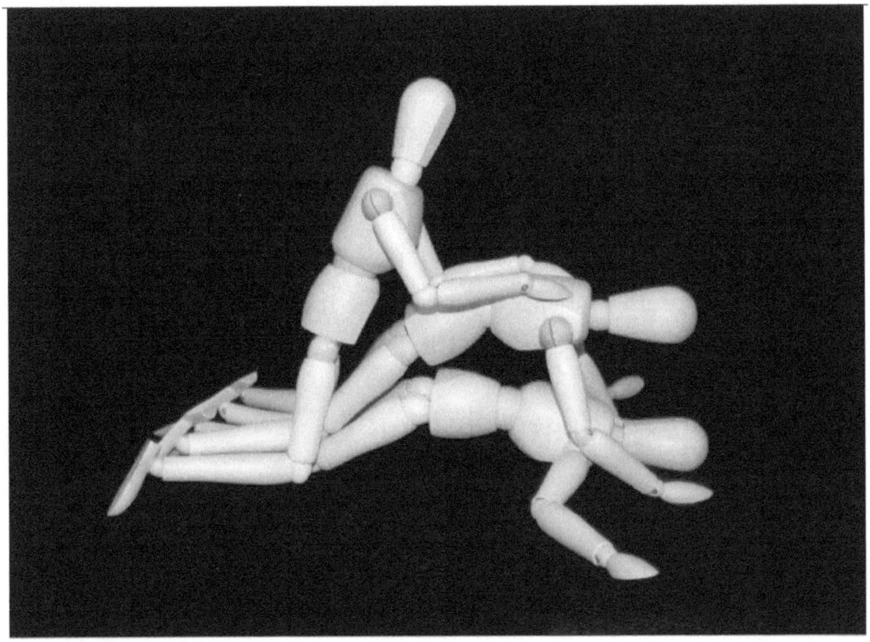

Position Description:

This positions requires two women and one man (or a strap on dildo sporting woman). If you don't have this type of makeup in your threesome, you are just going to have to skip this one and wait until you do.

To start this position, one of the women lies on the bed. She arches her back, but keeps her legs fairly close together (just wide enough to offer access to her pussy is perfect).

Now, the second woman climbs on top of her. She doesn't fuck her or anything like that. Instead, the second literally climbs on top of her and spreads her legs wider than the woman she is lying on. She arches her back to match the woman's she is lying on.

She should not be lying perfectly even with her. Her vagina should be positioned right above the bottom woman's tailbone if this is to work out right.

The man now approaches the pile of women from behind. From his point of view, he is now looking at two women, perfectly positioned and eager to be penetrated from behind. The man now has his pick of which woman to fuck and is free to go back and forth between the two. Lucky bastard!

Ease Of Position: Moderately Difficult

Depth Of Penetration: Shallow to Average

Good For Female Orgasm? No

Downsides:

The women are not in a terribly comfortable position. Depending on their weight and body compositions, the position may not be maintainable for too long. If you are the man you should keep this in mind.

Upsides:

The women are in a flush, body to body embrace. They are able to kiss each other's necks and feel each other's bodies. This is highly intimate. For the man, he is living out one of his fantasies. He is large, in charge and has his choice of which woman to fuck first. It's like he found a magic lamp on the beach!

Notes On This Position:

Let's be honest here. This position is a bit of an artificial one. The women would have little incentive to assume this position if they were not doing so to let the man live out one of his biggest fantasies. With all that being said, however, that does not mean that his position is without merit. The simple fact that this allows a man to live out one of his biggest fantasies ensures that it has a place in this book.

If you have decided to reward the man in your life with a girl on girl threesome, for whatever reason, make sure that you included this position. Heaven can wait! He will have already found paradise on Earth.

Doggystyle Double Penetration

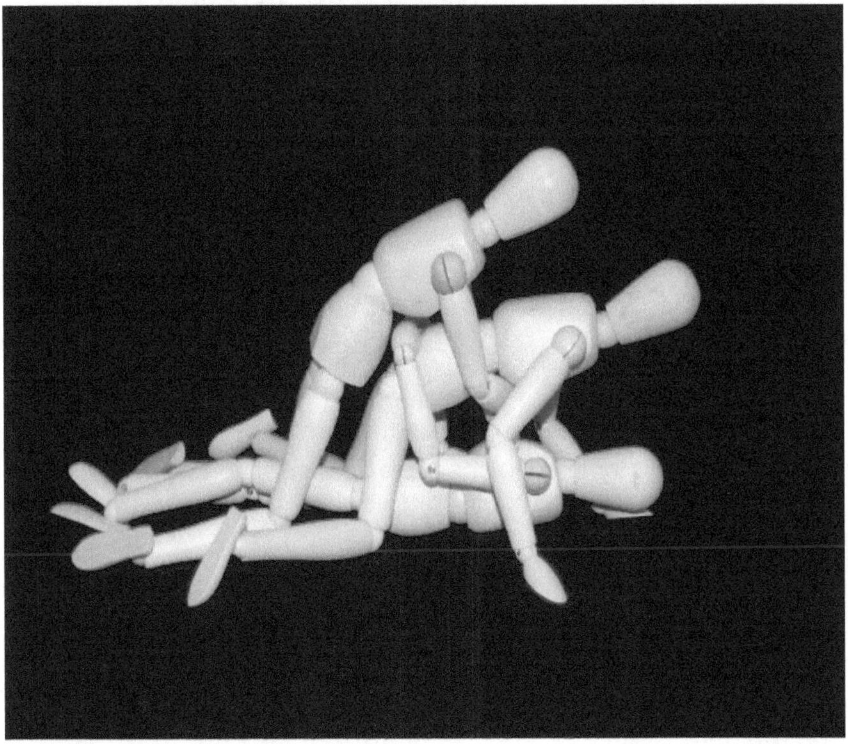

Position Description:

Double penetration positions require that a woman be involved. As such, to perform this position, at least one member of the threesome must be female.

To enter into this position, one of the male (or female with a strap-on dildo) lies on the bed. The woman who is to be penetrated climbs on top in the cowgirl position and places his cock inside of her vagina. In this position, the man on the bottom must have sex with her vaginally or things don't line up.

Now, the second man approaches her from behind and penetrates her anally.

Ease Of Position: Easy

Depth Of Penetration: Vaginal - Average, Anal - Deep

Good For Female Orgasm? No

Downsides:

In this position the man on the bottom has very little range of motion and cannot control penetration very well.

Upsides:

There is a lot of body contact here and a lot of closeness. The woman feels close to them men and at the same time completely dominated by them. There is lots of kissing, sucking, caressing and even hair pulling and biting if the action get hot.

Also, this position is very natural. It is really just combining to comfortable, easy twosome positions into one red hot threesome position.

This is a very intense sexual position for the couple to try.

Notes On This Position:

The man on the bottom, like I said, does not have a lot of range of motion as far as penetration is concerned. As such, he should focus on applying pressure into her vagina with his pelvis. This will increase stimulation for her. You, as the bottom man also are in charge of keeping her busy with kisses. Get in there and make sure her lips are busy. This will heighten her pleasure and yours.

The man that is penetrating her anally should also be gentle. It is easy to get carried away with anal sex and it can get too rough quickly. Start gentle, and as the three of you grow comfortable, she can tell you to increase speed or force, but wait for her invitation. You are a gentleman after all, even if you are fucking her in the ass.

Missionary Double Penetration

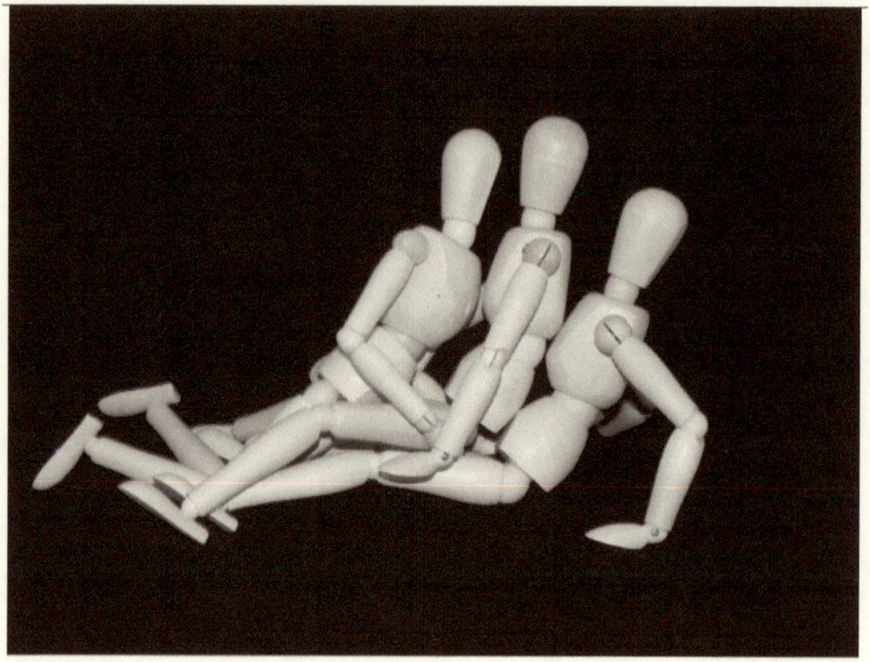

Position Description:

Again, as with all double penetration positions, this position requires at least one member of the threesome be a woman. The other two members can be real men, or women equipped with strap-on dildos.

One partner of the threesome begins this threesome by lying on the bed with an erect penis pointing up. The woman then sits on his penis and he penetrates he anally. It is important that the man on the bottom penetrates anally or the position will not work.

With one man's penis already inside her, the woman then spreads her legs and plants her feet on the bed. In this position, the second man can now take position between her legs, on his knees to penetrate her vaginally.

Ease Of Position: Easy

Depth Of Penetration: Deep Anal, Average Vaginal

Good For Female Orgasm? No

Downsides:

The man on the bottom has the full weight of the woman and a good part of the weight of the second man on him. This can be a little uncomfortable, but it is more than manageable. This also means that he is not in position to do any moving. As such, for any in and out movement, anally speaking, the woman is going to have to do the work. However, since she has the weight of the other man on her, her movement is restricted too.

Upsides:

Since this position puts the woman in control of the depth of the anal penetration, it can be considered a more comfortable position to engage in this novelty act.

Notes On This Position:

Double penetration is definitely a novelty act. It is a pretty unnatural sex position that is generally only found in porno movies. However, just because it is a novelty act does not mean that it has no place in your threesome. It is actually a lot of fun to carry out a novelty act. You will most likely laugh and smile at the same time you are enjoying the sexual sensation as well.

The Taco Buffet

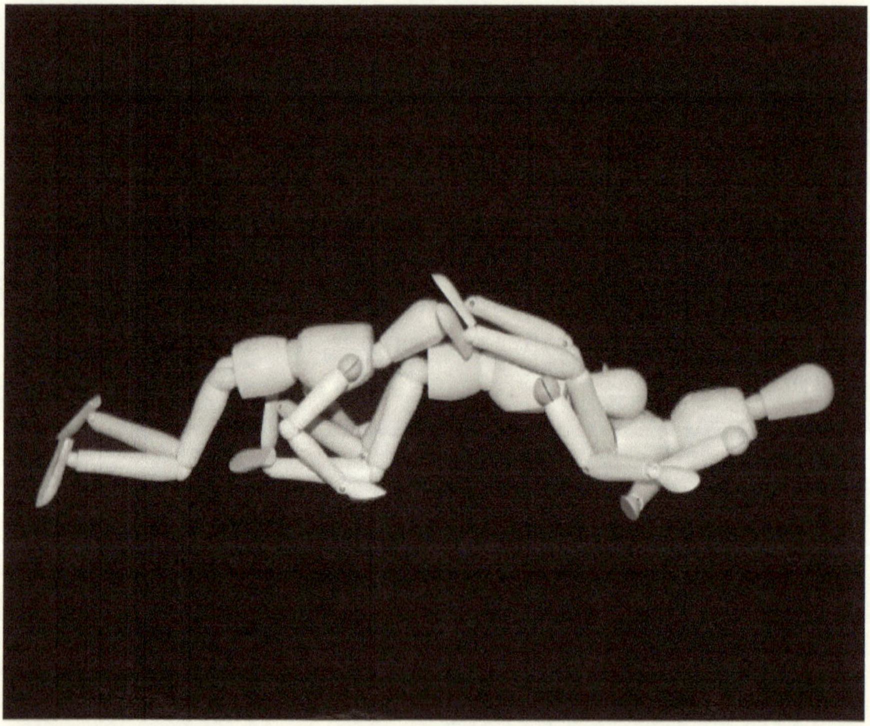

Position Description:

This position requires two women to be in the threesome mix. Just an FYI.

The first woman lies on the bed on her back. She spreads her legs and the second woman begins eating her pussy, in a four point stance.

Then, the third member of the threesome (man or woman) assumes a four point stance behind the second woman and and then begins eating her pussy.

This can continue indefinitely, and the two women can swap positions.

Ease Of Position: Moderate

Depth Of Penetration: N/A

Good For Female Orgasm? Yes and No

Downsides:

The person that is eating the pussy of the woman in the four point stance can get a stiff neck and cramps if this position goes on for a while.

Upsides:

Women don't get their pussies eaten enough. This is true in a threesome as much as it is in a twosome. This position takes care of that problem and sets aside a lot of time for the ladies to enjoy and get pleasured.

Notes On This Position:

For female orgasm, this position is marked "Yes and No". This is not a typo. Instead this is written to indicate that this position is great for female orgasm for the woman lying on her back. The woman on all fours will not be in a great position for clitoral stimulation. This can be corrected by having the man or third woman lie on the bed as well and the woman on all four can allow them to slide under her, between her legs so she can sit on their face. In this way, she too can be in a great position for orgasm, depending if that is the goal.

Daddy's Choice

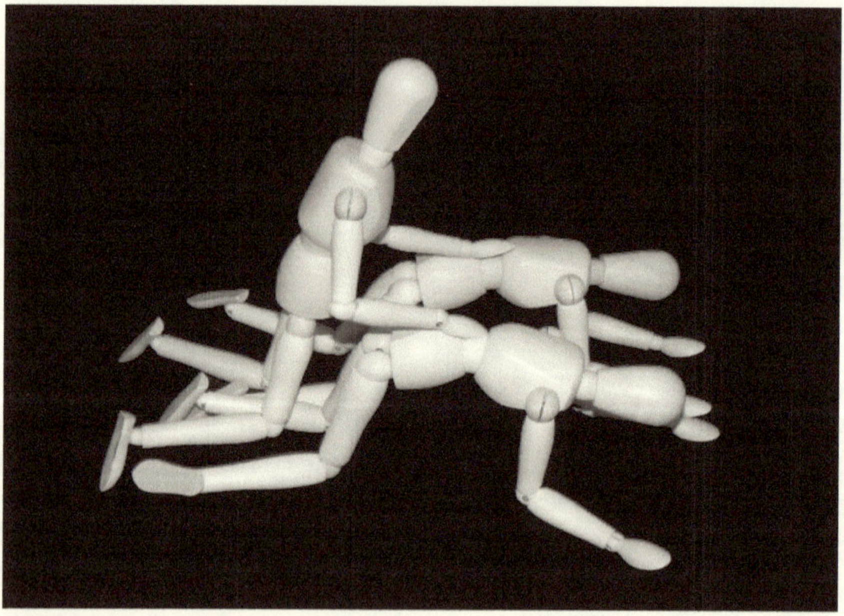

Position Description:

In this position, two of the threesome participants assume a four point stance. The lucky third member of the threesome can now penetrate the other two at their pleasure and go back and forth.

If anal sex is going to be had everyone involved should observe proper hygiene procedures. Nothing that has been inserted into an anus should be inserted into a vagina under any circumstances. This can cause medical problems.

Ease Of Position: Easy

Depth Of Penetration: Deep

Good For Female Orgasm? No

Downsides:

This position has two of the partners looking away from the third. Although they can interact with each other with kisses and eye contact, they cannot actually interact with the penetrating partner. This lowers the intimacy of this act significantly.

Upsides:

There is a fantasy, dominance aspect to this position that is a big turn on to a lot of people. One of the partners, the penetrating one, is king of the world. They are blessed with the choice of which of their partners they are going to fuck and how long, even going back and forth. This is a huge turn on.

Notes On This Position:

This is the position that you and your girlfriend give to your husband on his 35th birthday. He will feel like the king of the world and will not believe his luck. The two of you can kiss while he is going back and forth between fucking you. This will only add to his excitement. The visual stimulation is off the chart for him and you may be surprised how turned on you get watching him, balls deep in another woman, even more when she is making eye contact with you.

The Lucky, Lazy Man

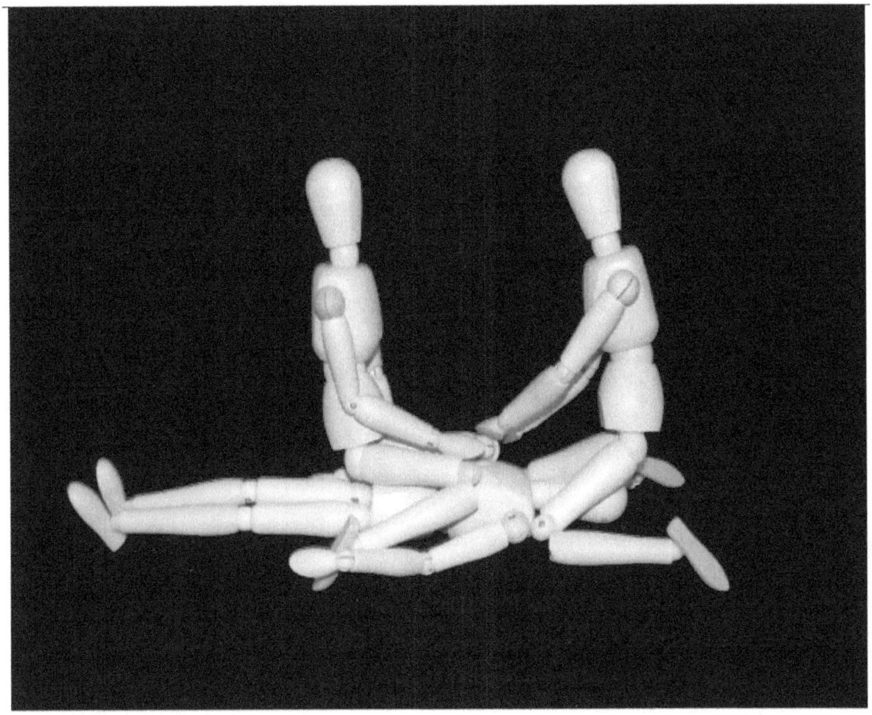

Position Description:

This position really only works in an MFF threesome, for the record.

The position begins by having the man lie down on the bed, face up. The first woman sits on his cock in the "Cowgirl" position that was described earlier. The second woman then sits on his face in the manner that was also described earlier.

As you can see, this is really just a compound sexual position that is made of two basic sexual positions.

The women also can change up this position by choosing to face away from each other or towards each other, or one of each. If they are facing each other they have the option to engage in foreplay activities.

Ease Of Position: Easy

Depth Of Penetration: Average

Good For Female Orgasm? Yes

Downsides:

In this position the man does not get to see anything. As men are highly visually motivated this can be a problem. However, the plethora of physical stimulation as well as the sights and sounds of this particular sexual act should more than make up for any loss.

Upsides:

In this position, the women are able to each receive one on one attention from the man. There is no necessity for any sort of lesbian behavior. This can be a plus in a threesome where the women are uncomfortable with any sort bisexuality, that is until things get more warmed up.

Notes On This Position:

This position is a great one for your first MFF threesome and is one you should not forget. It has a lot of advantages. One that is not readily appreciable is that the women are very much in control of the tempo of the sex. This can help to prevent an overly excited man cumming to fast at the thought of being with two women at the same time.

If the woman that is sitting on his cock is inclined to orgasm, she has two choices. The woman sitting on his face can stimulate her with a small vibrator until she orgasms. She can also face his feet and do the same or can even use her fingers.

If the woman that is sitting on the man's face is desirous of an orgasm, she really should face away from he cock and go down to a four point stance. This way, her clit will be in a perfect angle for him to apply the most amount of stimulation.

The Attendant

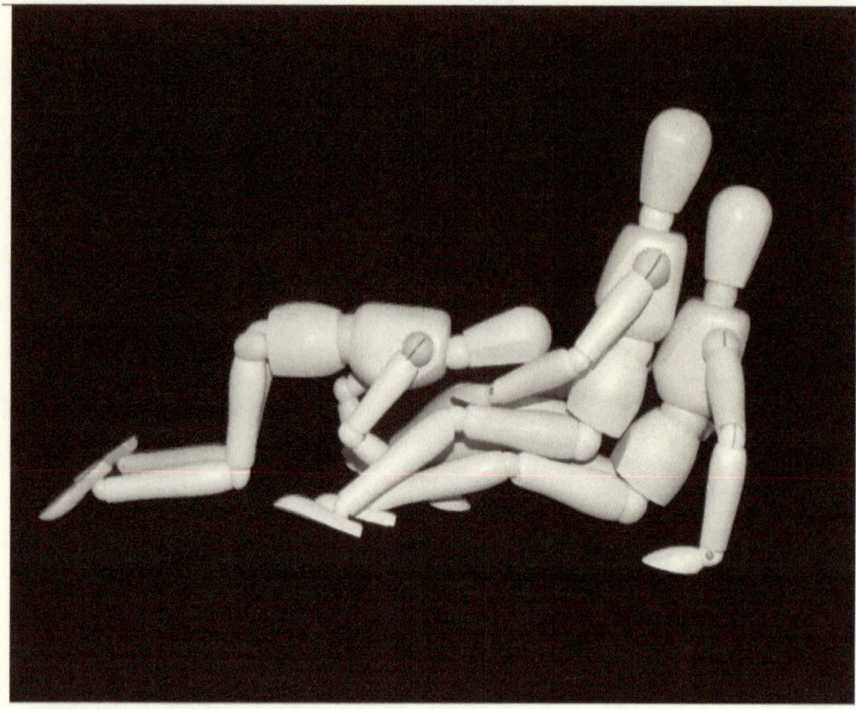

Position Description:

In this position, two of the partners engage in intercourse, either vaginal or anal. The penetrating man lies on the bed with his legs straight and closed. The person who is being penetrated (man or woman) then sits down on his penis and inserts it inside them. Once the penis is inserted, the penetrated partner places their legs on the outside of the penetrating man's. They then commence intercourse.

This is where the third person comes in. They assume a four point stance and place their face between the legs of the penetrated partner. Here they are in a position to perform oral sex on both people who are having intercourse. In essence, they are attending to their needs while they fuck.

If a woman is being penetrated either anally or vaginally, the attending partner will be in a perfect position to stimulate her clitoris. If on the other hand the penetrated partner is a man, the attending partner can give him a blowjob at this point. The attending partner can also interrupt intercourse and perform oral sex on the penetrating man as well or they can instead focus solely on foreplay style oral sex on his balls.

Ease Of Position: Moderate

Depth Of Penetration: Moderate

Good For Female Orgasm? Yes

Downsides:

It takes a little effort to assume this position, but that is really the only downside. Once the position has been entered into, it is a lot of fun for everybody.

Upsides:

This sexual position is particularly intense. There is a lot going on here and the visual for the attending partner is a lot of fun too. Also, if a woman is the penetrated partner in the intercourse part, she is in for a real treat. She is being penetrated by a real penis at the same time she is being given intense oral sex from her other partner. This can result in a powerful orgasm indeed.

Notes On This Position:

This position is very versatile in the context of a threesome. It can work with two men and a woman, two women and a man, three men, or even three women with a strap on. This makes it a very popular go to when three horny people get together.

You can also not overlook the fact that in this position, there is quite a bit of show going on. A big part of the fun in a threesome is watching other people have sex. This does that, but also lets the attendant participate as well. Next time you have a threesome of any kind, give this one a try!

The Sinful Missionary

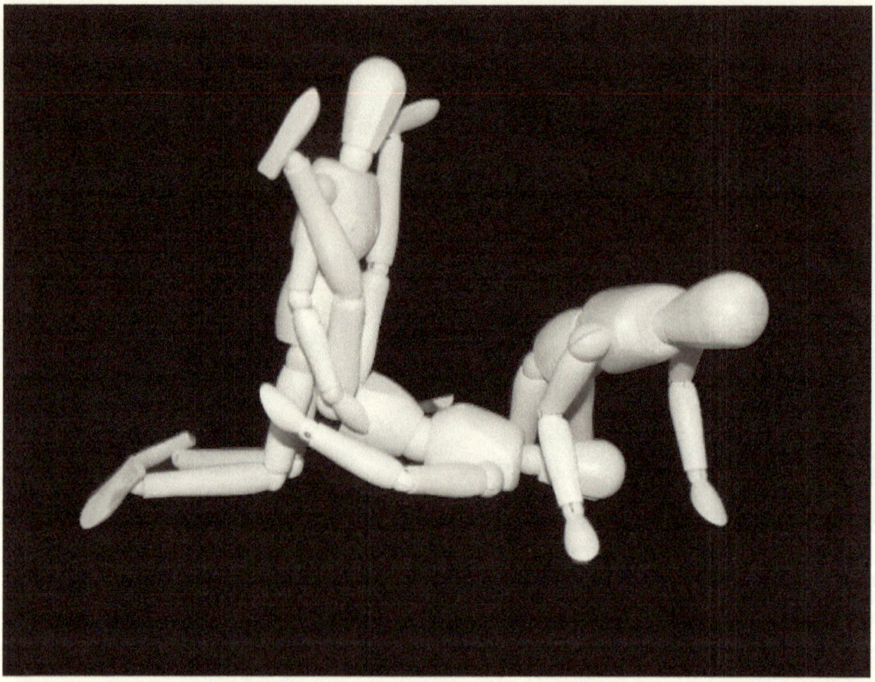

Position Description:

In this position, one member of the threesome lies on the bed. They lift their legs and allow a second member to penetrate them. Again, the penetration can be either vaginal or anal. The penetrating member of the threesome can even lift their hips for deeper penetration like is shown in the picture.

At this point, the third member of the group, a man, assumes a four point stance over the mouth of the person being penetrated. At this point, the penetrated partner can then give him a blowjob while he watches the other two engage in intercourse.

Ease Of Position: Easy

Depth Of Penetration: Average

Good For Female Orgasm? No

Downsides:

There is a lot going on in this position. The penetrated partner is sliding in and out and the penetrated partner is keeping their balance. At the same time the penetrated partner is having to focus on the blowjob they are giving. This means that this position is not good for female orgasm.

Upsides:

There is a lot going on in this position. That is what makes it appealing. There is a lot of sexy action to watch. There is also something for everyone. Someone is getting fucked. Someone is getting sucked. And two people are getting to do some fucking of some kind. Also, everybody is getting to watch everybody else and there is good face contact.

Notes On This Position:

The only threesome type that this position does not work for is three women. In that position, one of the women would have to be sucking on a strap on dildo of some kind and that is pointless. However, for any other combination of three horny people, this one will work. If three men are involved in the threesome, the penetrating man can also jerk off the penetrated man for even more fun.

There is also no reason that a woman cannot play the role of the penetrating partner. All they need to accomplish this is a strap on dildo. There will not be any direct stimulation of her pussy or clit other than what is afforded by the design of the strap on that she is using.

The Sinful Missionary – Version 2.0

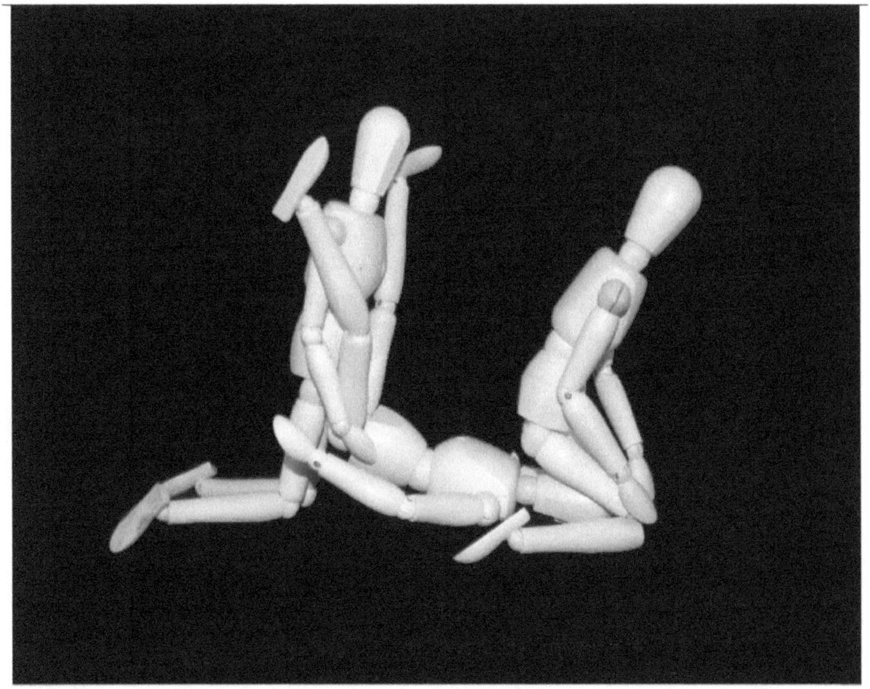

Position Description:

This position is identical to "The Sinful Missionary" except that instead of the penetrated partner performing a blowjob on the third partner, the third partner sits on their face. This person should be a woman. In this position, the penetrated partner can now eat her pussy.

Ease Of Position: Easy

Depth Of Penetration: Average

Good For Female Orgasm? Yes and No

Downsides:

Just like with the first version of this position, if the penetrated partner is a woman, she is not in a position to receive any type of clitoral stimulation.

Upsides:

Just like in the first version of this position, there is a lot happening. Everyone is getting attention paid to their bikini zones and is fucking or licking or being licked. This means that everyone is involved in the action. It also means that there is a lot to watch.

Notes On This Position:

The woman who is having her pussy eaten has a choice to make. She can either face into the action and watch the intercourse at which point her clit becomes less accessible to her partner, or she can face away from the action and really make it easy for her partner to pleasure her clit. If she faces away she is much more likely to have an orgasm, but will miss out on some of the visual fun.

Just like the other version of this position as well, this position works in most threesome combination. Three woman can be involved as long as one of them has a strap-on dildo. Two men can easily participate in this threeway as long as one of them is the one being penetrated. Lastly, and most easily, two women and a man can perform this act very easily if one woman is happy to be penetrated and eat the pussy of her other lover at the same time.

The 69 Assistant

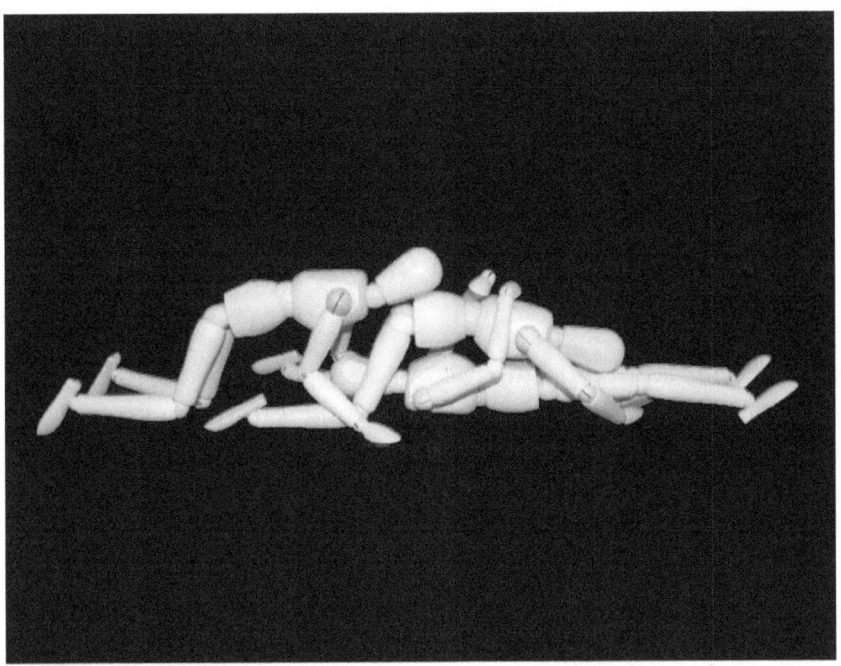

Position Description:

In this position, two of the partners engage in a normal Spirit of '69 position. Although the partner on top does not necessarily provide oral sex. This position is intended for their pleasure only so the option is theirs.

The third partner then assumes a four point stance behind the top partner in the '69 and begins to provide oral sex to their ass. In this way, the top partner is receiving oral stimulation to both their genitals and their anus simultaneously from both of their partners.

Ease Of Position: Easy

Depth Of Penetration: N/A

Good For Female Orgasm? Yes

Downsides:

One partner is directly licking another partners ass. This may be unpalatable to some people and thus will make this an undesirable position.

Upsides:

This position focuses the attention of two partners on the third completely through oral sex. This is intense, sexually speaking, and is very intimate. It is also a thrill to solely be the attention of two lovers, simultaneously.

Notes On This Position:

It cannot be understated how much of a turn on it is to be the sole object of attention of two lovers at the same time. This is something that many people will never even thought of until they are overwhelmed by the pleasure it can deliver. This position should definitely be used on any women involved in a threesome. They will love the attention and the pleasure until they cum.

This position is possible with men in the top position as well. Although, a blowjob is much harder to give from below. Instead, gentle, non-goal oriented oral sex should be given as foreplay.

Fantasy Double Blow job

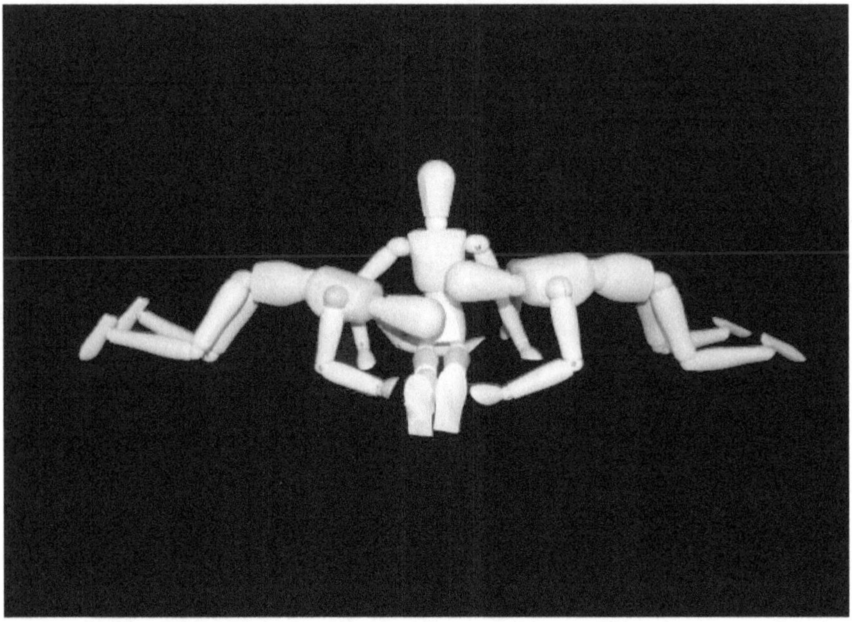

Threesome Type: MMF, MFF, MMM

Position Description:

One of the men (if there's only one, he's the lucky one) lies on the bed in the seated position. This also works on a couch for convenience. At this point, the other two partners take up positions on either side of him. From the side, both partners come in and engage in simultaneously giving him oral sex.

Ease Of Position: Easy

Depth Of Penetration: N/A

Good For Female Orgasm? No

Downsides:

This is a very lopsided sexual position, especially for a threesome. One partner is getting all of the attention and the other two are doing all the work. This can leave the two performing the act feeling a little ignored. If you are the lucky guy getting this kind of attention, you better make sure that you make it up to your partners by lavishing attention back on them.

Upsides:

Well as far as threesome fantasies go, this is one of the highest and most common among men, especially heterosexual ones. The idea of having two women (or a woman and a man) giving a simultaneous blowjob is about as good as it gets. This position, is the one that makes men try and have threesomes with two women in the first place. A definite must do for him.

This can also be a fun team building sharing exercise for the two giving the oral sex as well. They have to work together as a team to make sure that he receives all the pleasure he deserves. Group activities often bond people together. If the three of you are a little awkward at first, this is a good breaking the ice position.

Notes On This Position:

Obviously a man's cock can only be in one mouth at a time. This means that the two people performing the oral sex are going to have to share and coordinate. Take turns doing the actual sucking. There are a few options. Here are some examples of sharing:

- One sucks, then stops and the other takes over
- One sucks while the other provides some hand stroking
- One sucks while the other provides oral stimulation to the shaft of the penis or the balls, perineum, or even anus

Remember to share. It will foster a good environment of play, openness and fun!

Double Pussyeating

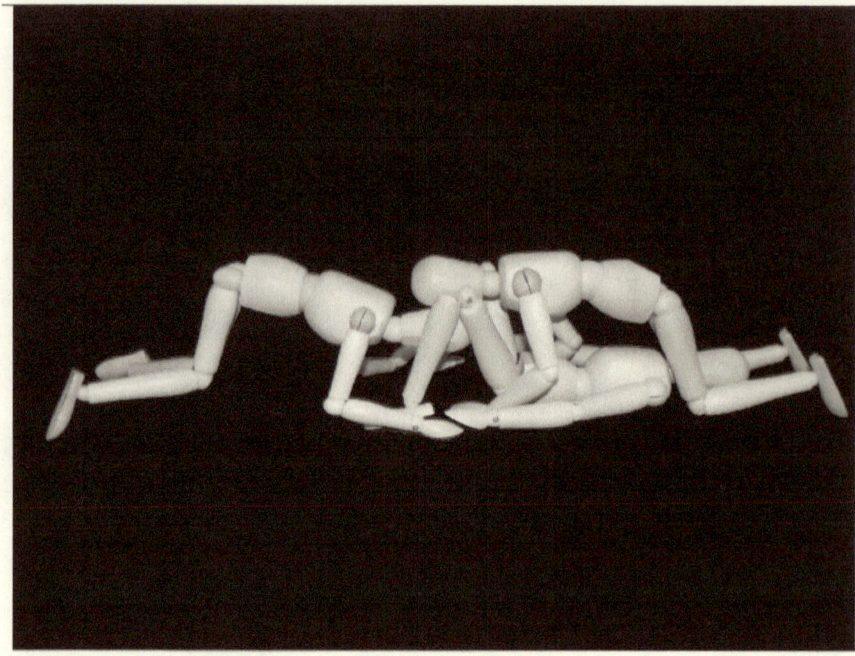

Position Description:

This is the female equivalent of the "Fantasy Double Blowjob".

One of the women (if there is more than one) lies down and spreads her legs like she would for the "Standard Pussyeating" position. One of her partners then lies between her thighs and prepares to eat her pussy. Her other lover, however, climbs on top of her in the 69 position. Now both of her lovers are able to orally stimulate her.

The woman whose pussy is being eaten also has the option to reciprocate oral sex to the partner above her. However, this is entirely optional and should have a non-goal, "I just want something in my mouth" theme to it.

Ease Of Position: Easy

Depth Of Penetration: N/A

Good For Female Orgasm? Yes

Downsides:

There aren't any appreciable downsides to this position other than the woman who is getting her pussy eating having someone else's genitals in her face. However, since she is letting them go down on her, that is probably actually a plus.

Upsides:

This is a way to make one of the women in a threesome feel great! The world stops and suddenly everyone is paying attention to her and her orgasm alone. Her two lovers are there only to lavish attention and pleasure on her. This is what she has been waiting her whole life for!

Notes On This Position:

Although there are not any real downsides to this position, there are some small hurdles that are caused by the discrete nature of a woman's pussy. When two people are going down on a guy, his cock is out there for everyone to put in their mouth and there is a lot of surface area to accommodate tongues and lips. This is not the case with a woman's pussy. The clitoris is much smaller and can be neatly tucked away, so the two people trying to lick her pussy are also going to have to work together, but in even better coordination than the "Double Fantasy Blowjob".

First, the person who is not in the 69 position is going to need to do all of the fingering. If the person in the 69 position with the woman tries to, they will actually block the woman's clit. Not good! So the person not in the 69 needs to take care of that.

Either one of the two partners can lick, suck, and tantalize the clitoris all they want, but only one person on the clitoris at a time. There is no sharing like the double blowjob. Space is too limited. Now if you don't have face time with the clit, that does not mean that you are useless. Au contraire! Instead, you need to be focusing on playful licking and kissing. Think tummy, thighs, feet, pussy lips, ass, perineum or breasts. Anyone of these areas loves to be tongue tickled while the clit is getting some attention. Trust me she will never tell either of her partners to stop.

So take your time, share and love her in a way she will remember for the rest of her days.

Swashbuckling Swordfight

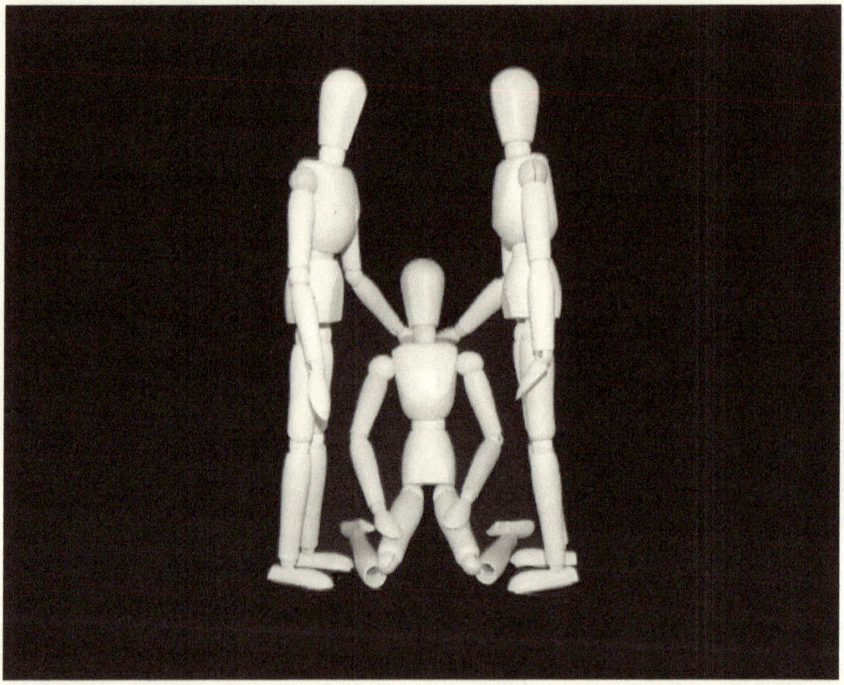

Position Description:

This position requires two dicks to get sucked so there must be at least two men in the threesome.

In this position, one of the partners gets down on their knees and gives blowjobs to the other two male partners.

Ease Of Position: Moderate

Depth Of Penetration: N/A

Good For Female Orgasm? No

Downsides:

While they are kneeling on the floor, the person offering the blowjobs is on their knees. This is fine for a while, however, if this act goes on for an extended period, this can become uncomfortable. To help deal with this problem it is courteous for one of the men who is getting oral sex to provide a pillow for the giver.

Upsides:

There is a lot of stimulation here for the two men. First, each of them is getting their cock sucked. This in itself can be a lot of fun. However, they are in a very good position to watch the other man get his cock sucked as well. This can be a huge turn on if the men are sharing a wife or boyfriend. As always, part of the fun of a threesome is getting to watch the other partners in action.

Notes On This Position:

In addition to having two cocks to suck the person on their knees has a lot of responsibilities. First, they need to make sure that they are doling out their oral favors in a manner that is fair and attentive to both of their lovers. This is one of those positions that can make one of the men feel left out. So, make sure you are really doing a good job of going back and forth.

One tip to help alleviate this problem is to keep a hand on both cocks. Both should always be stroking. That way, wither man is getting some attention even if it isn't your mouth.

You also have the option of trying to put both cocks in your mouth at once. This can be a playful but of oral fun and you should give it some thought. It also depends on your lovers. This sort of action involves penis to penis contact. This can push the bounds of sexual comfort for some men. If you're not sure, better just to forget this part.

In pornos, this is the classic "cum on their face" position. It is very possible this is what the men who are getting the oral sex will assume. As always with cumming on or in things, all three of the lovers should be on the same page before the act begins. Don't be afraid to set boundaries. Good times are based on strong boundaries.

Lastly, for the men, they are in the standing position. Plenty of men can lose their balance while they are cumming. To avoid this issue, this act is best performed in front of a bed frame of a wall that they can lean on. That way, when the time cums, they can surrender and enjoy the moment without winding up in a pile on the floor.

<u>Fuck Or Suck?</u>

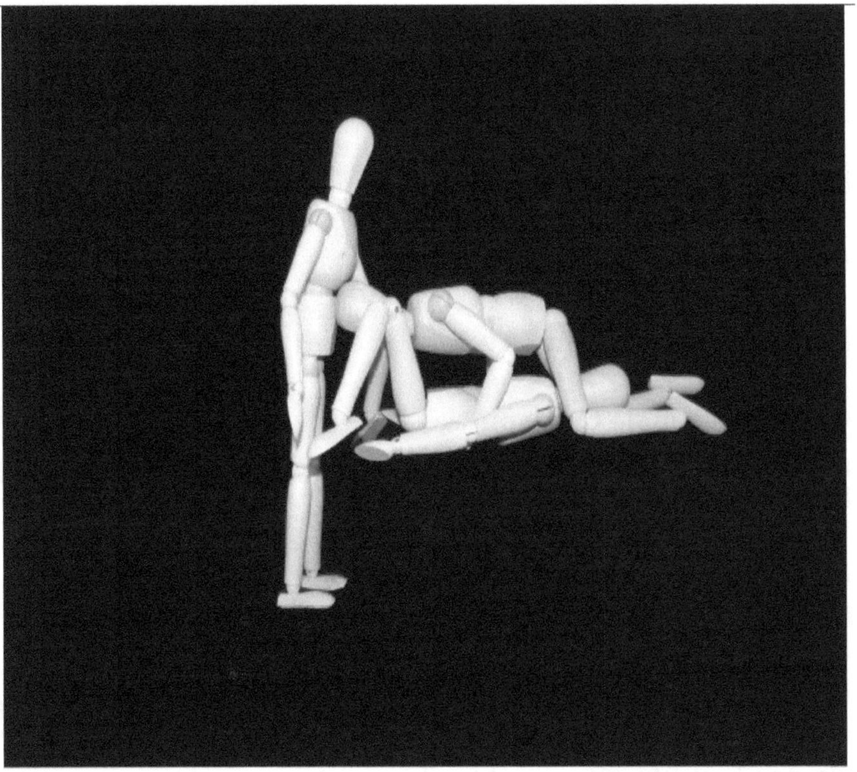

Position Description:

In this position, one of the partners lies on a surface that is about waist high. A high bed, a counter top, or even a sturdy dining table will suffice.

They spread their legs and a second partner penetrates them. Penetration can be either vaginal or anal, depending on the gender of the partners or personal preference.

The third partner then straddles the first partner in a classic "69" position. They are now in to suck the cock of the penetrating partner when they interrupt intercourse. The penetrating partner is now in a position to go back and forth between oral sex and penetration at their discretion.

Ease Of Position: Moderate

Depth Of Penetration: Average

Good For Female Orgasm? Yes

Downsides:

In this position, as always when a part of it is the "69", somebody's face is usually right up close to someone's ass. This can be a problem for squeamish lovers. Also, some women are just really not into having a guys undercarriage right up in their face either. If the penetrated partner is a woman that fits either of these two categories, you might want to skip this one.

Upsides:

For the penetrating partner, it doesn't get much better. How often has he fantasized about fucking someone and getting his cock sucked at the same time. Well, today is his day and he is in charge of what happens. Only he can decide which type of stimulation he is to receive. The only trouble is he may have trouble picking and sticking to one and may just wind up going back and forth – a lot.

Notes On This Position:

For the two in the "69", there is no reason that you can't cum too. The guy doing the penetrating will sooner or later, so you might as well get in on the action.

Two options exist. Since you are both in a good "69" position there is the option that you can orally pleasure each other to orgasm.

Now if a woman is being penetrated, especially vaginally, it can be hard to get in there at the right angle to give her an orgasm. In that situation it is best to fall back to our old friend the small vibrator. That will do the trick no problem. This too will work for the person in the top of the "69" as well.

The Pileup

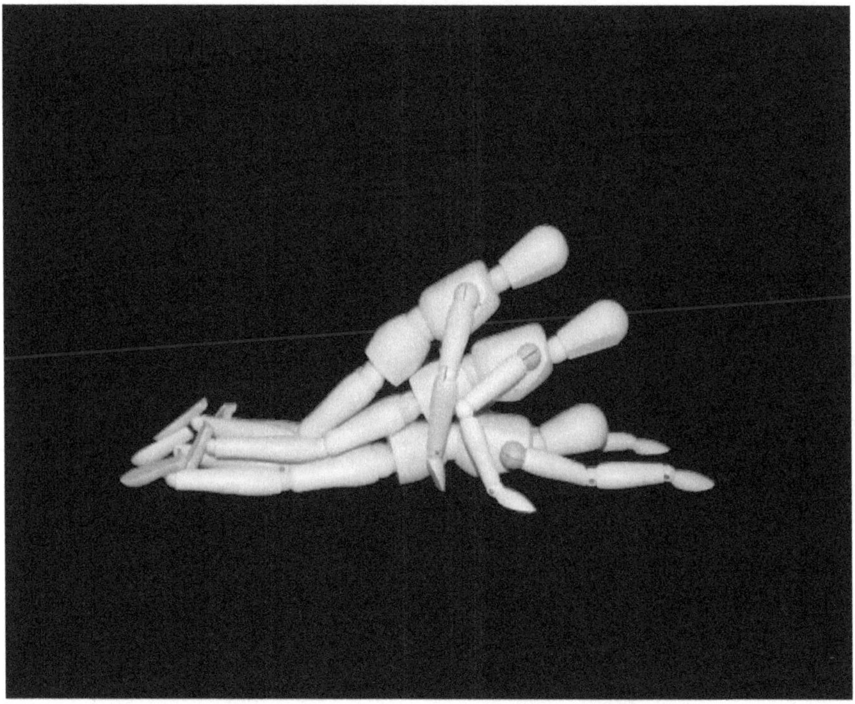

Position Description:

In this position one of the threesome partners lies on the bed. They arch their back and spread their legs. If the person is a woman, both her pussy and ass are now exposed. If the person is a man, his ass is exposed for anal sex.

A second partner then climbs on top of partner lying on the bed and penetrates them either anally or vaginally.

Lastly, the third partner climbs on top of the fucking couple and penetrates the second partner. At this point, one partner is being penetrated, one partner is being penetrated at the same time they are penetrating someone else and a third partner is just penetrating.

Ease Of Position: Difficult

Depth Of Penetration: Average

Good For Female Orgasm? No

Downsides:

The person on the bottom of the pileup has the weight of two other people on top of them. This can be uncomfortable depending on the weight of the other two partners and the surface that they are on. For this reason, you need to make sure that the bed is good and plush.

Also, on this position, there is not a lot of room for people to move their hips for deep penetration. Instead, participants in this position, need to rely more on subtle hip motions and gentle, connected penetration.

Upsides:

This position does not rely on deep, vigorous penetration for the fun. The fin comes from three people sharing full body contact and being inside one another. This also affords the opportunity for lots of touching, caressing, rubbing and kissing. These activities really make this one a lot of fun.

Notes On This Position:

This position seems to imply that there needs to be at least one man in the mix. This is definitely not true. As long as there is a t least one strap-on dildo at the party, this act can be enjoyed my MFF, or even FFF threesomes as well. Even if there isn't a real penis, you all can still enjoy this one.

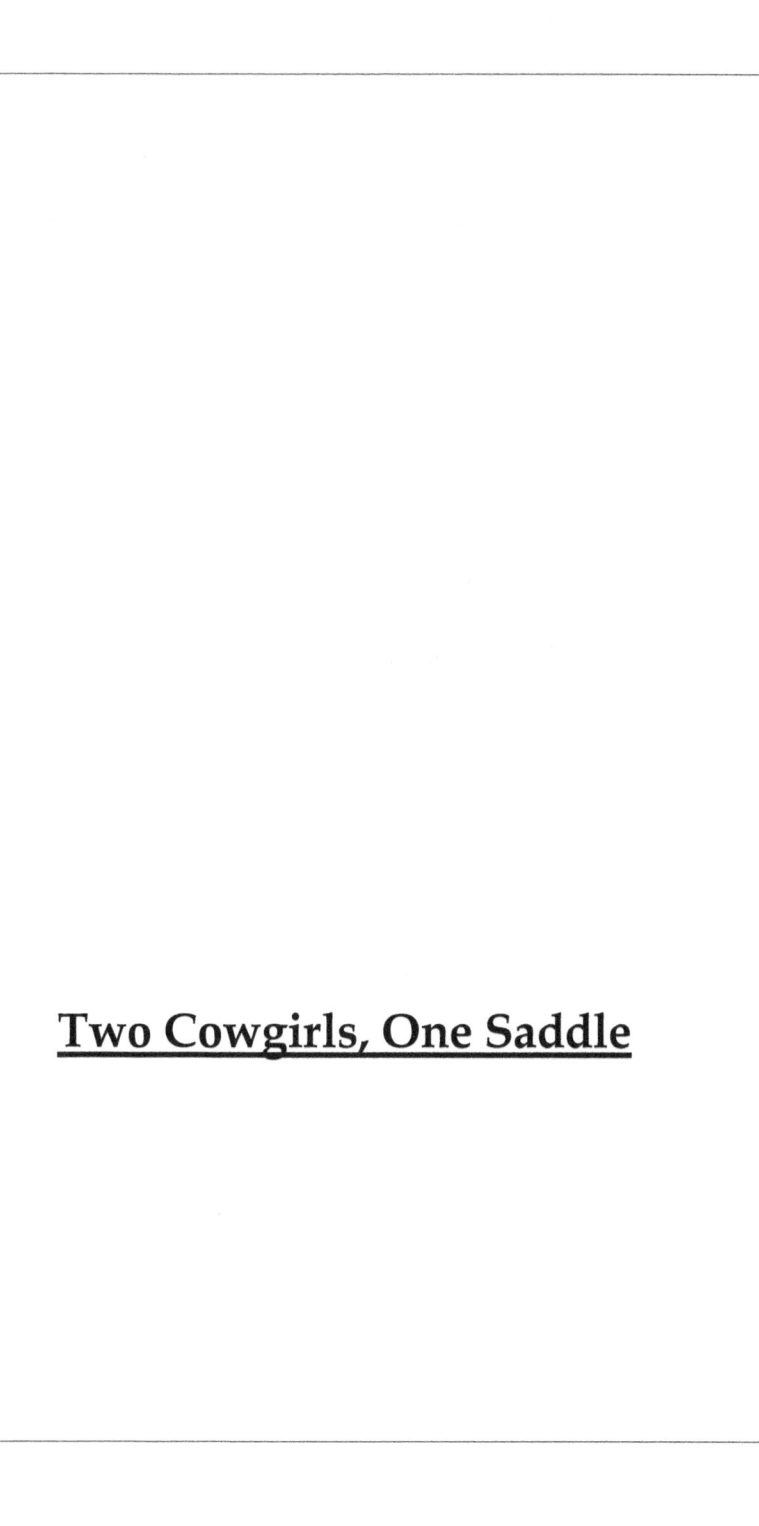

Two Cowgirls, One Saddle

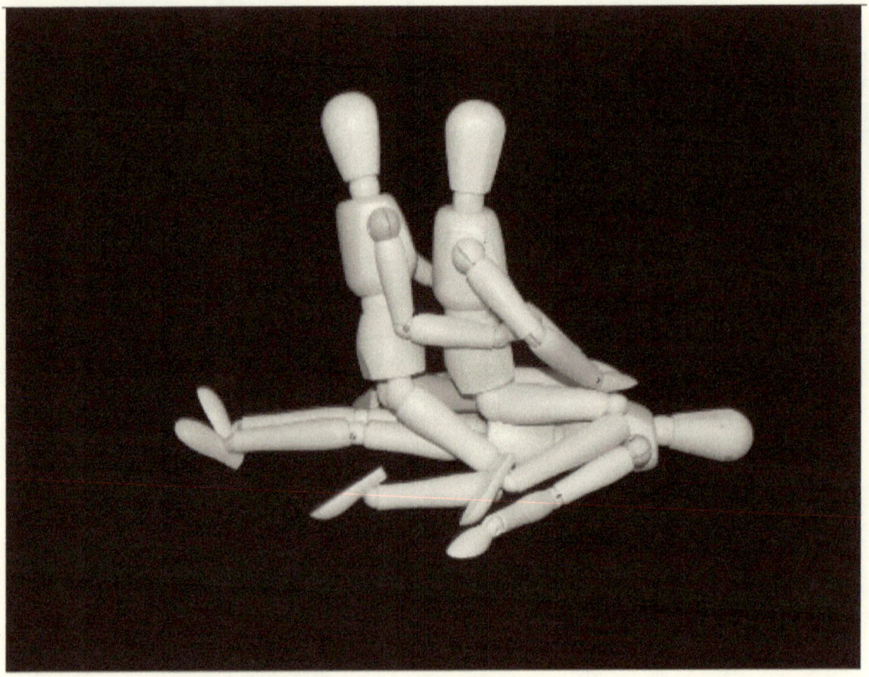

Position Description:

In this position, one of the partners lies on the bed. A second partner then straddles them in the classic "Cowgirl" position and is penetrated. This penetration can be either vaginal or anal depending on the sexual makeup of the threesome and the preferences of the individuals involved.

With two partners of the threesome already engaged in sex, the third member straddles the legs of the penetrating partner and sits down. They are now in a position to lavish attention on the penetrated partner.

Ease Of Position: Easy

Depth Of Penetration: Average

Good For Female Orgasm? No

Downsides:

In this position, the third partner (the one behind the penetrated seated partner) is not getting any attention from anyone. This is only a potential downside and is one that can be eliminated easily enough by making sure they get attention from both partners later.

Upsides:

The partner that is being penetrated is in the position to receive stimulation from both of the pother partners. In the one case, they are looking down on a lover that is inside of them. There is strong eye contact, and there can even be kissing if they bend down.

On the other hand, they are receiving tender, affectionate attention from the partner behind them as well. They are able to lavish kisses on their neck, back and even lips with some neck arching. If the penetrated partner is female, there is also lots of hands to caress her breasts and ass as well.

Notes On This Position:

As I pointed out when discussing the downsides of this position, the person in the back of the saddle is not getting a lot of attention. This can take the threesome into a twosome plus one ignored lover. Everyone needs to make sure that this person is still part of the fun.

One of the easiest ways to accomplish this is simply to take turns. One person gets to sit on the cock for a while, then you switch it up. This will make sure that everyone is in on the action and feels involved.

Side By Side - Threesome Style v1.0

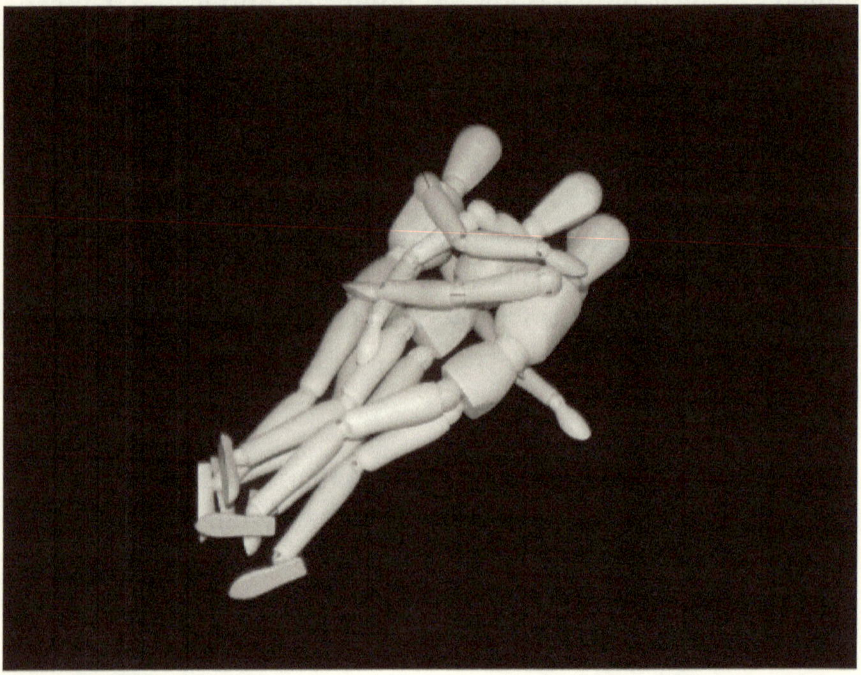

Position Description:

In this position, one of the partners lies on the bed. A second partner lies down behind them like in the "Side by Side" twosome position. The partner in behind penetrates the first partner. These two then engage in lovemaking. The third partner then lies in front of the penetrated partner. They are now in a position to make out with the penetrated partner, or just as importantly, they can now watch the other two fucking. This is true pleasure.

Ease Of Position: Easy

Depth Of Penetration: Average

Good For Female Orgasm? No

Downsides:

The one downside to this position is that one of the partners is not in on that making out. However, they are involved in the intercourse. This keeps them involved in the sex act.

Upsides:

This position is a great resting position and it is very intimate. All of the partners are close, and are in a position to be in physical contact with one another. This can be very tender. Also, the physical demands of this position are low for everyone. This should be a go to position for the trio after hours of horseplay and wild fucking. Everyone can catch their breath and relax for a bit.

Notes On This Position:

Due to the fact that this position is a good resting one, it often finds its place at the end of the threesome once everyone is a little tired. All too often, however, people overlook this positions importance in starting a threesome.

An example will help.

Imagine you and your two friends have been out clubbing all night. You've had a few drinks and people are feeling pretty good. Well, the cab drops you all off at your place. No one really wants to go anywhere but to bed to catch some sleep. Only one problem. There is only one bed. No worries. We can all pile in there. No one is squeamish. The three of you aren't lovers yet, but you're not prudes either. You all pile into bed.

Well, this position comes naturally enough to three people in bed. It's really just a passion bomb waiting to go off. You, as the one who wants to get things going only has to make a move on one of the other people in the bed. If they reciprocate, it is easy enough to quickly welcome the third person into the action. You're all close and touching anyway, why not start fucking? In this situation, a full on fantasy threesome will quickly follow.

So, remember that one when you've got two partners you are trying to seduce simultaneously. Clubbing, then back to your place, "Hey, my bed is big enough for us all. No worries.", then a little seduction and you're on your way to a night of fantasy sex you have previously dared not dream of.

Side By Side – Threesome Style v2.0

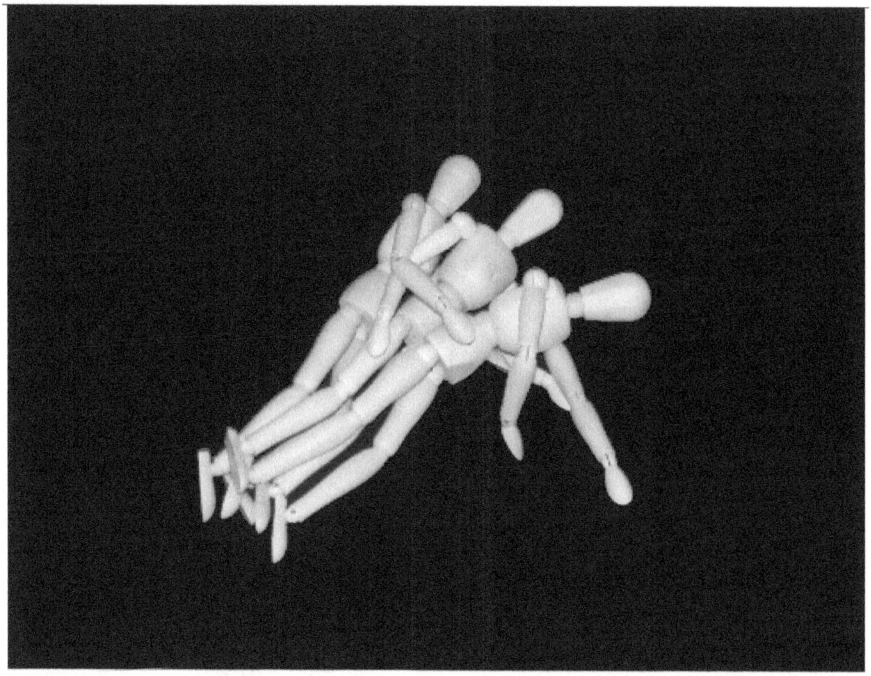

Position Description:

You can think of this position as a modified "Pileup" with the participants lying on their sides. This will help put thing in perspective a bit.

One partner lies on the bed on their side. It doesn't matter if it is the left or the right.

A second partner then approaches them from behind (also on their side) and penetrates them. Now, the penetration as is common in this book, can be either vaginal or anal. Also, depending on the sexual makeup of the group, the penetration can be with either a real penis, or a strap on dildo, as needed. Lots of possibilities and lot of options.

Lastly, the third member of the menage a trois, approaches the second partner and penetrates them. Again, this can be either anal or vaginal and can be either a real cock or a strap-on dildo as well.

If the position is assumed correctly, two partners are penetrated and two are penetrating. One lucky partner is getting both!

Ease Of Position: Easy

Depth Of Penetration: Average to Shallow

Good For Female Orgasm? Difficult

Downsides:

Like most positions that involve double penetration, there is not too much room for deep penetration, hip movements. This means that the penetration is gentle. To some, this can be a problem.

Also, in this position there is no face to face, intimacy building eye contact.

Upsides:
OK. So there is no deep penetration or face to face contact. That does not mean that this position is not intimate. There is lots of full body contact, including penetration. The threesome is literally connected into one body. There are lots of hips to caress and backs of neck to lavish with kisses.

Also, like any and all sexual positions that are on their side, this position is a great resting position. The pace is slow, but the sex is still great.

Notes On This Position:

This position is a lot of fun. It is close, and tender and soft and is something that any threesome should give a try.

Round Robin Oral Sex

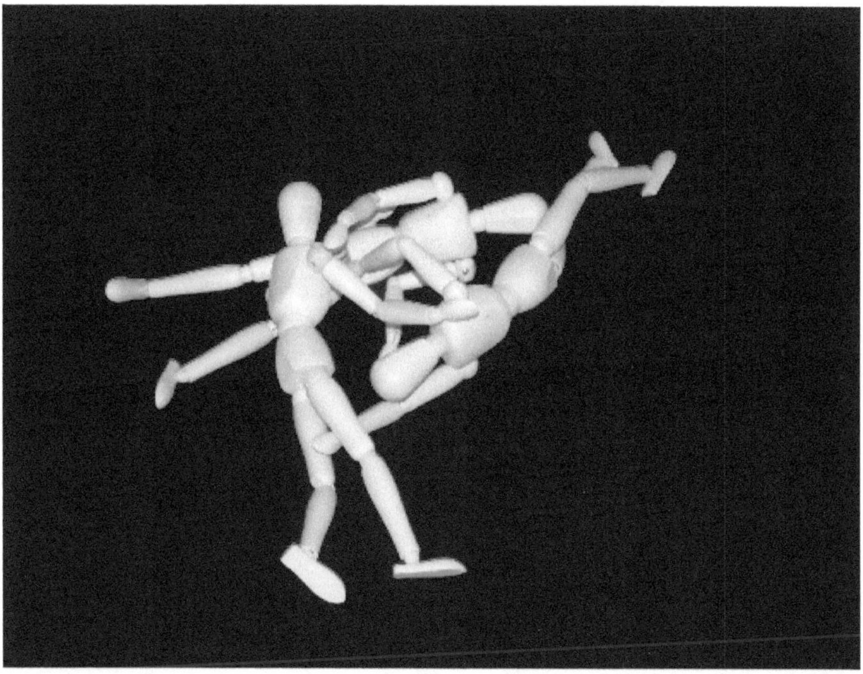

Position Description:

So many of the positions in this book involve penetration in one manner or another, as well as an oral sex component. This position on the other hand is a purely oral sex position.

The flow of the act is fairly basic. One of the partners lies on the bed, a second partner then lies down with their head in the first partners lap in a perpendicular manner. The second person then begins to give oral sex to the first.

The third partner then lies down with their head in the lap of the second, again, in a position that will permit them to give the second partner oral sex.

Now, for the coup de grace, the first partner then repositions, still while receiving oral sex from the second partner, to a position that will allow them to give oral sex to the third partner.

If you have followed the instructions correctly, everyone will be both getting and giving oral sex. It should also be pointed out that this position works in any gender combination.

Ease Of Position: Easy

Depth Of Penetration: N/A

Good For Female Orgasm? Potentially

Downsides:

Life is about making choices. We often have to give a little to get a little. This is a good way to sum up this position. The truth of the matter is that in this position, none of the women are in a great position to get orgasm oriented oral sex. The angles just don't work out perfectly. That is the sacrifice that must be made for everyone getting their cake and getting to eat it too.

This is not to say that there cannot be orgasms with the aid of a small vibrator. There definitely can and this is something that is worth trying!

Upsides:

Just because this position is not at the right angle to make women cum orally, does not mean we need to throw the baby out with the bath water. This position is a lot of fun. Everyone is in on the action and the women's pussies get plenty of oral attention. This is a great way to make sure that any women are plenty wet before any penetration begins.

Of course, too, it is worth pointing out that the men are in a very good position to cum. This can be a really, really, fun position if the threesome is made up of three men.

Notes On This Position:

For couple who limit their group sex activities to oral sex only, this is one that you need to remember! It is intense, lots of fun and is full of visual stimulation. You may have to strain your necks a little to make all the pieces line up, but it is worth it in the end!

T-Boning Facesit

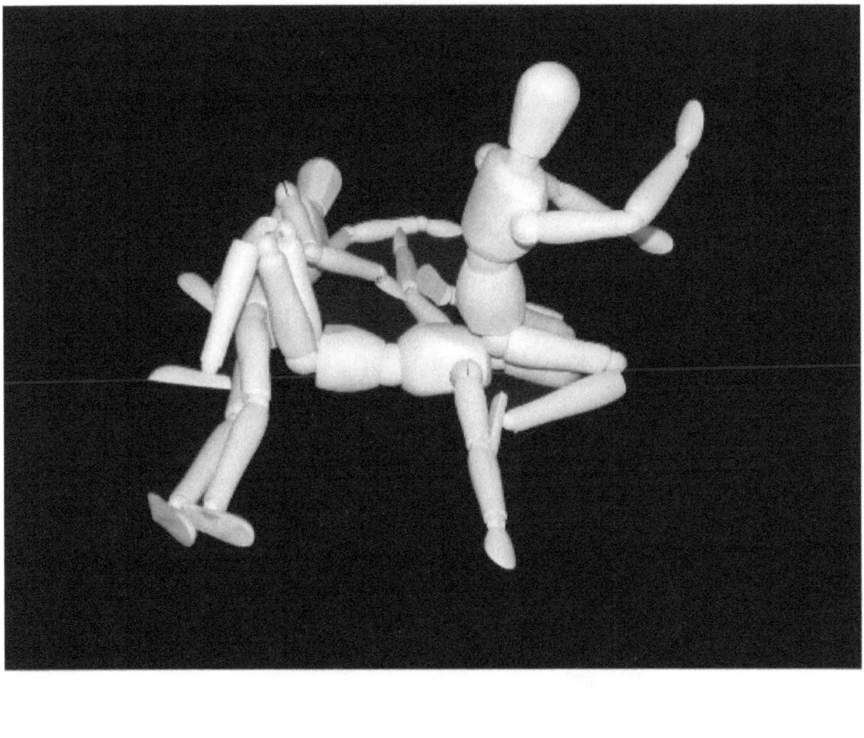

Position Description:

In this position, one of the partner lies down on the bed and lifts their legs into the air. They bend their knees and keep their legs in the air for a moment. A second partner lies perpendicular to them and penetrates them in the classic "T-Bone" position. At this point, the two engage in intercourse, either anal or vaginal.

The third partner, in this position, a woman, then sits on the face of the penetrated partner. The penetrated partner is now engaged in intercourse and is eating the pussy of the third partner.

Ease Of Position: Easy

Depth Of Penetration: Shallow

Good For Female Orgasm? Yes

Downsides:

Like with any oral/penetration combo, the person in the middle has a lot going on. However, unlike the other positions in this book that employ both oral and penetration, this one is much slower in tempo. The man (or woman with a strap-on) doing the penetrating is lying in a position that forces them to slow down. This largely negates the overwhelming stimulation that is so common.

Upsides:

Since the woman who is getting her pussy eaten is in the seated position, she , not the woman being penetrated is in control of movement. The woman who is doing the pussy eating really just lies there and acts as the stimulator. The seated woman has the responsibility of moving her clit where it will get the most attention. This also helps to take pressure off the penetrated woman and makes the stimulation and enjoyment much more of a group thing.

Notes On This Position:

Since this position spreads out the pleasure and stimulation, as well as the responsibility to keep things going, it is a really good starter position in the oral/penetration class. The slower tempo allows the threesome to learn to work together as a team. This in turn makes the faster paced ones much more possible.

Also, it should be noted that the woman who is being penetrated is in a great position to masturbate with either her fingers of a vibrator. The penetrating man, however, is not in a good position to offer her clit any stimulation. The angle is just no good. If she wants to cum, she is going to have to do the work

Missionary Double Penetration

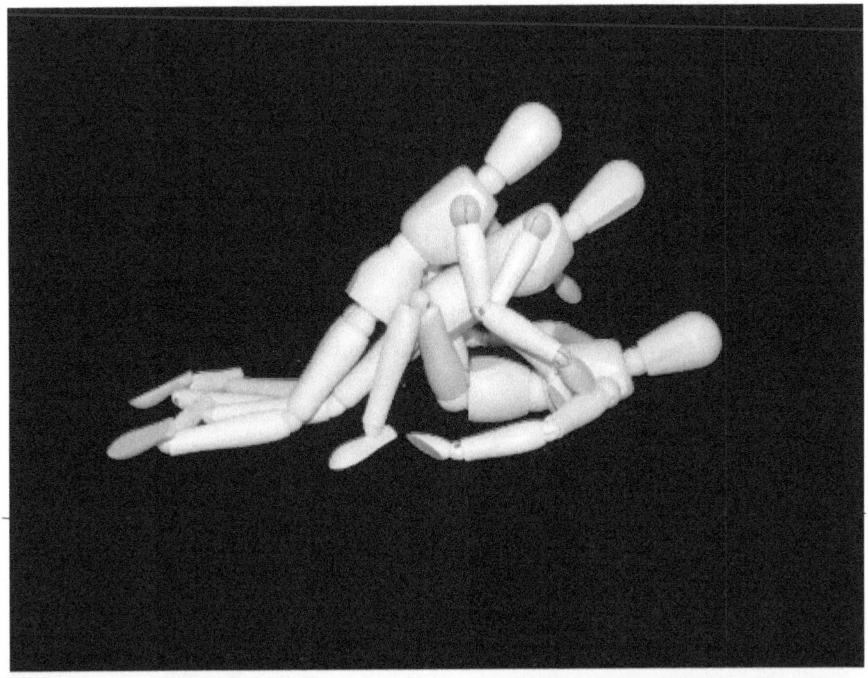

Position Description:

In this position, one of the partners (presumably a woman) lies on the bed and spreads her legs. A second partner, either a man or a woman with a strap-on dildo lies between her legs in the classic missionary position and penetrates her. The two then engage in face to face intercourse.

However, in this position, there is a twist. There is still a third person that needs to get in on the fun.

This partner (again a man or a woman with a strap-on dildo) then approaches the person who is doing the penetrating and penetrates them. If this is a woman with a strap-on, it can be vaginal or anal and the design of strap-on dildos will make this possible. If it is a man, then the penetration will need to be anal.

Ease Of Position: Moderately Difficult

Depth Of Penetration: Average

Good For Female Orgasm? No

Downsides:

The big downside to this position is the lack of range of motion. This position is similar to the "Pile" position in that only the person on top is free to move their hips. This means that the penetration, especially the two in the missionary position.

Upsides:

There is a lot of face to face and closeness in this position between the lovers. This allows for lots of kissing, nuzzling and caressing. This makes it a lot of fun.

Notes On This Position:

Unless there are some bisexual men in the threesome, this position is going to require some pre-planning. By this I mean that you are going to need to have some strap-on dildos handy. In all honesty, this is something that any free thinking, threesome desiring person should have handy anyway. Like so much in life, it's better to have it and not need it than to have it and not need it.

The Fluffer Blowjob

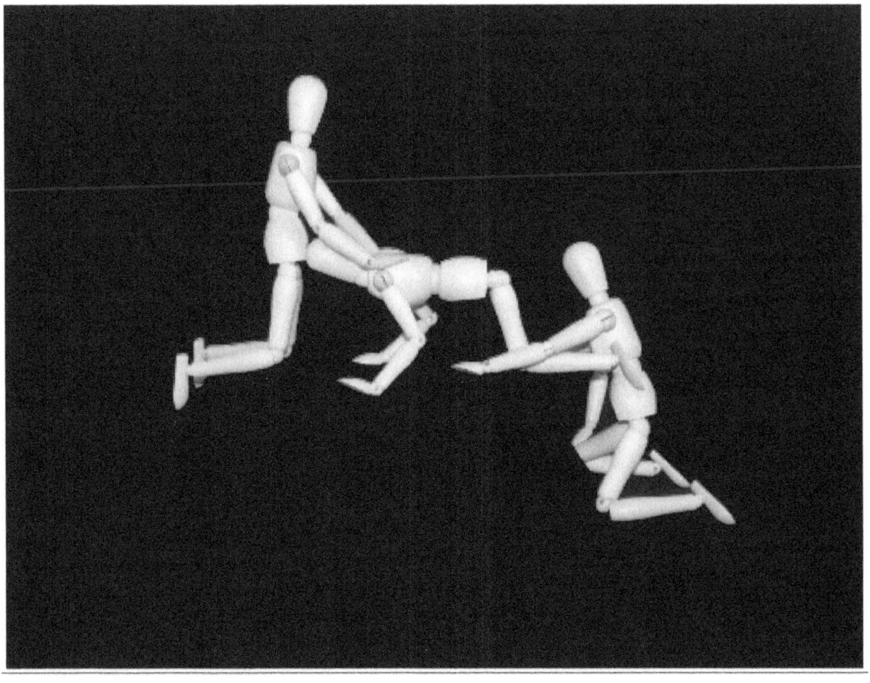

Position Description:

This is a blowjob position.

One of the partners assumes a position on the bed, on all fours. Another partner climbs on the bed in front of the first partner, on their knees. They place their cock (or even dildo) into the mouth of the partner on their knees.

Up until this point, this is simply a dominant blowjob as discussed in my first sexual positions book. However, we are going to add a twist.

The third partner now approaches the partner on all fours from behind and begins to give them oral sex. For convenience, this can be either on the bed, or they can be on the floor on all fours.

Ease Of Position: Easy

Depth Of Penetration: N/A

Good For Female Orgasm? Yes

Downsides:

There are no downsides to this position. Everyone is having a good time.

Upsides:

The person who is both getting and giving oral sex, is getting all of the attention. This is a good way to lavish attention on one of the partners if they have been neglected for a while.

Notes On This Position:

This position is called the "Fluffer Blowjob" for a reason. The person who is giving oral sex to the partner on all fours is doing so in anticipation of intercourse. The intention is for the partner who is getting a blowjob to stop and then begin to fuck the person who was blowing them. In reality, the partner giving oral sex to the partner on all fours is getting them ready for sex, or fluffing them.

This position has a lot of dominance and psychology at play. The person who is "fluffing" is acting as a servant to the other two and their sexual needs. This can be a lot of fun in wife or husband swapping scenarios, when a new partner is offered to a member of an established couple.

Undercarriage Double Team

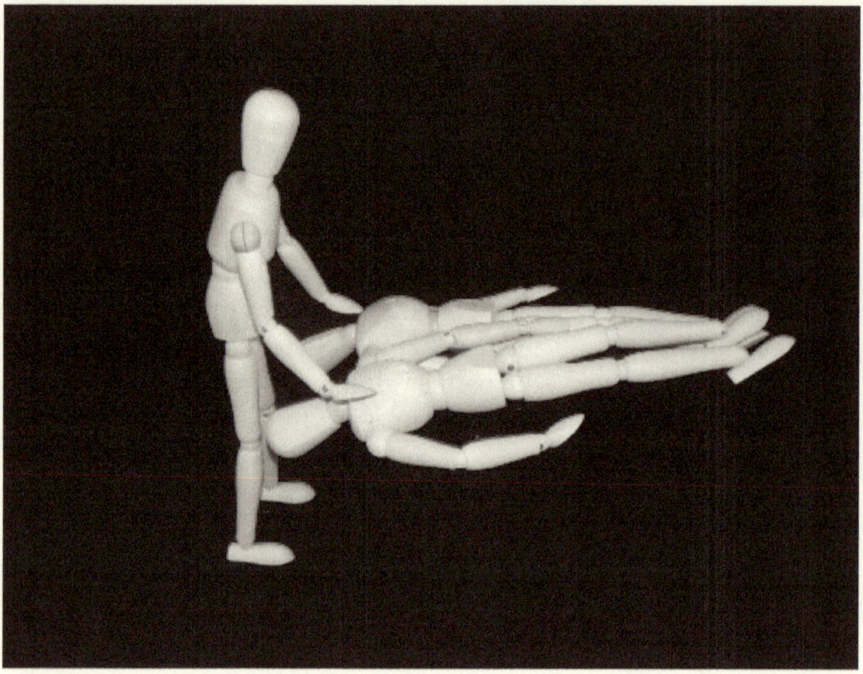

Position Description:

This is a blow job position.

The partner that is going to receive oral sex stands between the heads of the other two partners, who are lying face up on the bed. Their heads are hanging off the bed.

The two on the bed then lean towards him and can perform any number of oral sex techniques on this cock, balls, perineum and even anus, as a team.

Ease Of Position: Easy

Depth Of Penetration: N/A

Good For Female Orgasm? Yes

Downsides:

If the partners giving oral sex lie upside down for too long, they can get light headed. Also, if the man getting oral sex is pleasured to orgasm, he can easily lose his balance.

Other than these two minor problems, this position is a lot of fun.

Upsides:

This position is another feast for the eyes of the person getting oral sex. They are looking down on their two lovers pleasuring them and they have the full view of their lover's bodies as well. They are king of the world while the position lasts. This is the kind of position that you want to spoil your husband with when you surprise him with a threesome!

Notes On This Position:

The two partners lying on the bed are in no way limited to only pleasuring the standing lover. Quite on the contrary! The are in a very good position to either play with each other or themselves. They can easily cross over and manually stimulate each other with hands (either handjob or fingering) or they can also masturbate to orgasm themselves. A pair of vibrators will make this an explosive orgasm position for everyone. In almost every case, the man getting his cock sucked will on enjoy this position's more as he looks down on his two lovers not only sucking his cock, but masturbating to orgasm in anticipation of him fucking them to boot!

T-Bone Mouthfuck

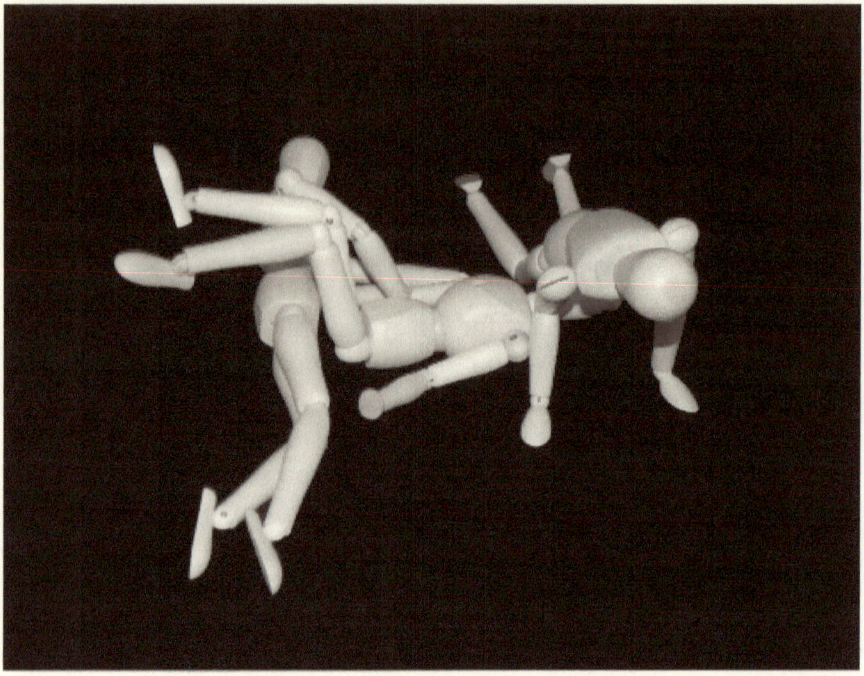

Position Description:

This position is only a slight modification of the "T-Bone Facesit". This version has one partner lying on the bed and being penetrated by a second in the "T-Bone" position. However, instead of having a woman sit on the penetrated partner's face, a man (or as usual a woman with a strap-on) then mounts their face. From there, they are able to fuck their mouth.

Ease Of Position: Easy

Depth Of Penetration: Shallow penetration, deep oral

Good For Female Orgasm? Yes

Downsides:

The main downside to this position is that mouth fucking can always go a little too deep and cause discomfort or gagging. The best way to combat this problem is, as always, for the woman to keep a hand on the cock she is sucking. This will give her control over his penetration and can act like a brake for any problems. Fortunately, in this position, the woman who is being penetrated has both hands free to control the oral sex.

Upsides:

The couple that is engaged in intercourse are engaged in a lazy, slow paced bit of sex. This makes this position a great resting position when they need to catch their breath.

Also, as is usually the case with T-Bone positions, the woman is in a great position to play with her own clit to orgasm. Always a big plus.

Notes On This Position:

With mouth fucking, you need to have a plan if the man who is getting his cock sucked is going to orgasm. The woman is not in a very convenient position to get up and spit if she needs to. So make a plan a head of time.

Double Coquettish Blowjob

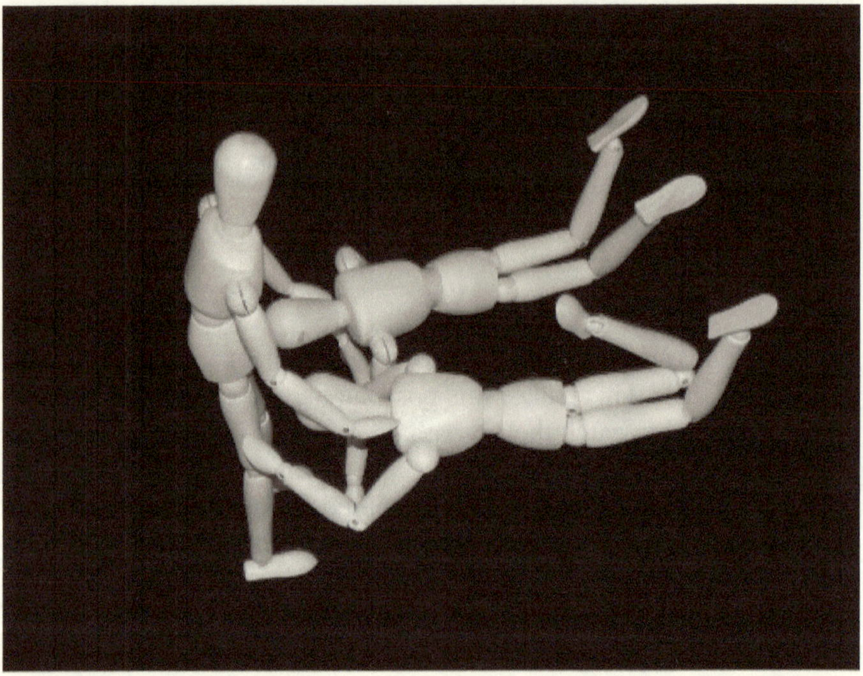

Position Description:

This is a blowjob position. In it, two of the partners lie on the bed face down and arch their backs. The third partner stands at the foot of the bed and allows them to pleasure him.

Ease Of Position: Moderate

Depth Of Penetration: N/A

Good For Female Orgasm? No

Downsides:

The angle that the two partners performing oral sex must contort too is a bit uncomfortable. Backs and necks are not designed to arc like that and muscles can become a little bit sore after a bit.

Also, if the man who is getting the blowjob reaches orgasm, as usual he may have trouble. He will have to choose between surrendering to the pleasure of the orgasm or maintaining his balance. A four poster bed will give him something to hang on to the help alleviate some of this problem.

Upsides:

The two who are doing the sucking are the ones in control of this act and they get to conspire to tease their lover. This can be a lot of fun for them and helps to bring the two of them together in the threesome.

Notes On This Position:

Since this position allows two partners to gang up on and tease the third with a blow job, it is a really good one to use if two women are a little nervous in the beginning of the threesome. It allows them to work to a common purpose which creates unity. At the same time, they are not in a position to look over each other's bodies. This can be a huge help in the beginning stages of a threesome when bashfulness can be a big impediment. By the time this act is over, they will be plenty horny and may even be to the point of making love to each other. Any speed bumps are happily in the rear view mirror at that point.

Doggystyle Lazyman Fuck

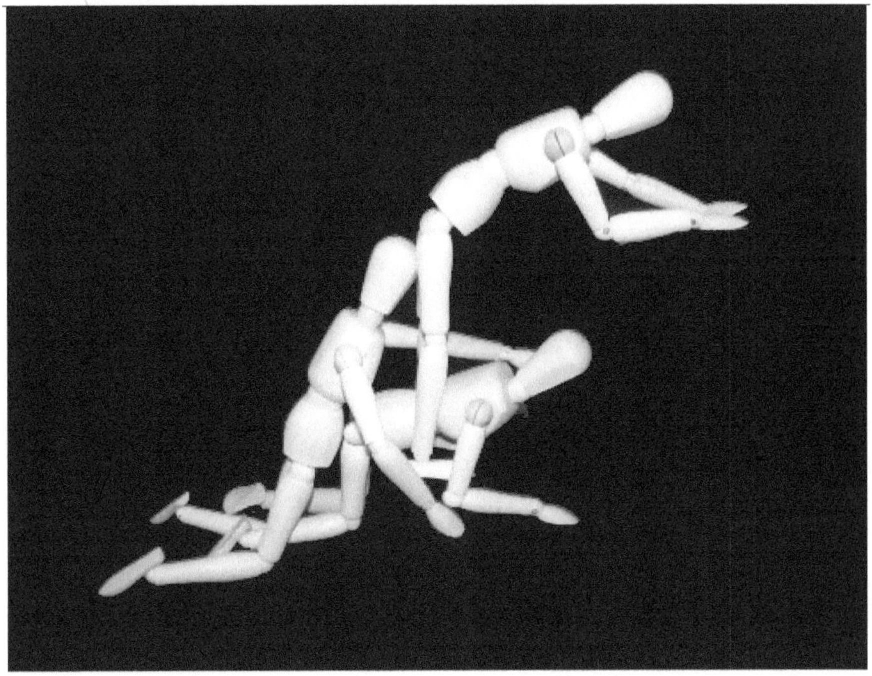

Position Description:

In this position, one of the partners assumes a doggystyle stance on the floor in front of a couch. Their torso should be on the sitting seat of the couch, but their knees should be touching the floor.

At this point, a second partner comes up behind them, also with their knees on the floor, and penetrates them. The two are now engaged in doggystyle sex on the floor in front of the couch.

This is when it gets fun! The third partner now stands on the couch above the first, penetrated partner. Their feet should be planted on either side of the torso of the first partner.

Now, from their position behind the first partner, the second partner can engage in oral sex on the third partner at the same time they are fucking the first. Awesome!

Ease Of Position: Easy

Depth Of Penetration: Deep

Good For Female Orgasm? No

Downsides:

The one big downside to this position is the need of a couch. This means that this type of sexual activity has to be undertaken in a location where the threesome won't be interrupted. Roommates and other people can walk in on you unexpectedly. This is the kind of position that you need a private living room to enjoy.

Upsides:

The best part about this position is that it is a lot of fun and it's easy. Everyone is in on the action, and everyone is comfortable. Also, the penetrating partner is getting completely overwhelmed with sexual stimulation. It is their lucky day for sure.

Notes On This Position:

This is a really nice, versatile position. For example, if it is more comfortable or more convenient, the penetrated partner can also roll over and be in missionary position. In this way, they actually get to watch the oral sex happening between the other two partner. That's a lot of fun for them and they get in on the visual stimulation.

Also, there is no reason on Earth that the penetrating partner cannot stand up and start fucking the other standing person. Unless there is a huge difference in height all of their bits should line up just right. They are then free to go back and forth.

www.ingramcontent.com/pod-product-compliance
Lightning Source LLC
Chambersburg PA
CBHW020306290526
45784CB00003B/1376
9781475015201